"This book is brilliant! With deep compassion, intelligence and humor, Dr. Huberman guides the reader through the often confusing and frustrating world of surgical weight management. He writes as both a learned psychologist and a best friend who is eager to support you in your journey. His unique insights and scientifically sound proposals are refreshing to encounter in a field where there has been so much misinformation. I will recommend *Through Thick and Thin* to every overweight patient in my practice."

BARRY LUBETKIN, PH.D.

Board Certified in Clinical & Behavioral Psychology (ABPP)
Director & Founder, Institute for Behavior Therapy

"*Through Thick and Thin* is an odyssey of personal and professional reflections on becoming and remaining thin. It explores body image, guidelines, pitfalls and zeniths of the journey through weight loss surgery. It will be both a bible and best friend for those considering or undergoing weight loss surgery, as well as those whose loved ones are starting that journey. This book goes above and beyond the usual medical jargon and diet practices—a great read."

BRADLEY SCHWACK, MD

Assistant Professor of Surgery,
NYU School of Medicine
NYU Langone Weight Management Program

"*Through Thick and Thin* is an outstanding, authoritative manual for anyone contemplating or having gone through weight loss surgery... Few professionals are as knowledgeable as Huberman in understanding the emotional journey that leads to candidates' massive weight gains, or the host of problems that may eventuate after surgery... The author approaches this sensitive topic as a consonant professional, but with a sense of humor that I have rarely seen in a book of this sort. His own personal struggles with lifelong weight issues become a story line...which allows the reader to easily connect with him and enjoy his humor and breezy style. I thoroughly enjoyed Huberman's book... *Through Thick and Thin* should be a must read for anyone contemplating weight loss surgery—for that matter, anyone who has lifelong weight issues in general."

STEVEN T. FISHMAN, PH.D.

Board Certified in Clinical & Behavioral Psychology (ABPP)
Director & Founder, Institute for Behavior Therapy

"Warren Huberman writes in a humorous but well thought out way, addressing the myriad of issues facing people on their weight loss journey. Speaking from personal experience, his rapport with the subject is unparalleled. He brings true insight into complex issues and gives people a real way of addressing problems. This book is a must have for everyone! We all know someone who has tried to lose weight. What we learn from the book is how we can all be better and more mindful to our friends, colleagues and family."

MARINA KURIAN, MD

Assistant Professor of Surgery,
NYU School of Medicine
NYU Langone Weight Management Program
Author, *Weight Loss Surgery for Dummies*

THROUGH THICK & THIN
THE EMOTIONAL JOURNEY OF WEIGHT LOSS SURGERY

THROUGH THICK & THIN
THE EMOTIONAL JOURNEY OF WEIGHT LOSS SURGERY

Warren L. Huberman, Ph.D.

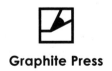

Graphite Press

PUBLISHED BY GRAPHITE PRESS

Copyright © 2012 by Warren L. Huberman

www.graphitepress.com

Front Cover Photograph
Copyright © 2007 by John Woodworth

LIBRARY OF CONGRESS CATALOGING-IN-PUBLICATION DATA

Huberman, Warren L., 1967–
Through thick & thin : the emotional journey of weight loss surgery /
Warren L. Huberman. — 1st ed.
p. cm.
Includes bibliographical references.
ISBN 978-0-9755810-9-4 (pbk. : alk. paper) — ISBN 0-9755810-9-0 (pbk. : alk. paper)
1. Obesity–Surgery–Psychological aspects.
2. Obesity–Surgery–Patients–Mental health.
I. Title.
II. Title: Through thick and thin.
RD540.H863 2011
617.4'3–dc23

2011042710

MIX
Paper from
responsible sources
FSC
www.fsc.org   FSC® C004071

PRINTED IN CANADA

First Edition

10   9   8   7   6   5   4   3   2   1

Acknowledgements

To Drs. Christine Ren Fielding, George Fielding, Marina Kurian and Bradley Schwack, and all of my colleagues at the NYU Langone Weight Management Program, for giving me the opportunity to do work that I love…

…and to Barrie and Dylan for giving me all the love I need to do my work.

Contents

Part I
Why Surgery?

Part III
Slip Slidin' Away

Part IV
Dealing With Others

Part VI
Moving Beyond Surgery

Appendices

Introduction

PERHAPS YOU'VE DECIDED TO PICK up this book because you're thinking of having weight loss surgery. Maybe you're still on the fence and are browsing this book while standing in the self-help aisle at your bookstore. Maybe you've had weight loss surgery and are struggling, or want to make sure that you don't struggle. Or maybe you want to learn ways that you can help a loved one who's contemplating surgery, or is facing some issues after having had surgery. In all these cases, this book will be helpful to you.

Weight loss surgery is a revolutionary and powerful tool to help folks lose weight and take control of their lives. However, it's a long journey and there's considerable work to be done beyond the operating room. Having worked with thousands of surgical weight loss patients, I can tell you that those who are most successful recognize that the surgery itself is only the beginning. In fact, many of my patients have shared that losing the weight and making the required dietary and behavioral changes surrounding eating was the easy part. Most people are either unaware of or completely underestimate how remarkable the psychological changes can be following surgery. It's often those psychological changes that enhance or hinder true success from weight loss surgery.

If you have already had weight loss surgery, congratulations! You've made one of the more challenging decisions in your life and hopefully you will be rewarded. If you're experiencing some psychological difficulties since having surgery, I'm confident that you'll find many of your concerns addressed in the pages to come.

If you're the person reading this book while standing in the self-help aisle of the bookstore, grab this book and run to the checkout line immediately! This is probably not the first time you've considered weight loss surgery and perhaps you're still not totally sure. Hopefully my book will answer many of your questions and help you make a more informed decision as to whether you're ready for weight loss surgery. Although this kind of surgery may not be appropriate for everyone, if you're one of the increasing numbers of people struggling with 100 pounds or more of excess weight, or have weight-related medical problems, it is unquestionably a method worthy of great consideration.

My Language

The only thing I ever wanted more than to be thin was to help people be happy. I'm sure the two are related. What you'll notice in the book are many efforts to keep things light, pun intended. (See I did it already!) Friends and colleagues tell me that, for better or worse, I write like I talk. I know of no other way and I really don't want to learn another way. I dislike political correctness because it dilutes the language to the point that we lose the meaning behind the message! Phrases like "big-boned," "large and lovely," "husky," and "plus-sized" are created as efforts to minimize judgments and make us feel more comfortable. But they don't always help. In fact, these phrases sometimes can be *more* critical and judgmental of others than simply saying "fat." When I use the word "fat," I'm referring to the size. It's not a character assassination, nor an insult. Unfortunately, our society has made the word "fat" the ultimate four-letter word.

Similarly, the word "obese" and the phrase "morbidly obese" refer to clinical levels of being overweight. These words have special meaning in the medical literature, and say nothing about why someone is overweight, or the causes of their weight gain. They are descriptive, no different than saying an orange is round and plump.

I want you to be entertained while you read, because I think it's the best way to learn. Rest assured that I am not poking fun at you. Rather, I am poking fun at the ridiculousness of the struggle to lose weight. I also like to poke fun at how irrational and stupid we humans can sometimes think and behave. Humor is a great tool and in my opinion is underused in efforts to help people learn. While you'll find that I use humor in large doses throughout the book, and speak in plain politically incorrect language, I make every effort to be sensitive to the difficulties faced by those who are overweight. The manner in which obese people are treated is not a laughing matter. If you read something that gives you a twinge, please don't take offense. Nowhere do I mean to insult or offend. I hope you come away a bit more informed along with a smile on your face.

My Mission

My mission was to write a book on weight loss surgery that takes the reader through the entire process, beginning with considerations prior to having surgery all the way to the complete physical and psychological transition following surgery. Each chapter was designed to address an important issue, based on my experience working with patients who have had surgery. In these pages you'll find the concerns and challenges patients bring to me after surgery. I've addressed a wide range of topics and I'm confident that you'll find much of the information to be quite useful. Hopefully, you'll find reading the book to be time well spent. I wish you the very best you on your journey.

—WLH

For Family, Friends and Professionals

I TRUST THAT YOU'LL FIND this book to be informative and helpful as you care for someone contemplating or recovering from weight loss surgery. If you're a friend or loved one of someone considering surgery, you no doubt recognize how much he or she has struggled with weight. As a professional, you've seen those struggles, challenges and concerns in your work with overweight patients. Perhaps the best way to utilize the information in this book would be to step into the shoes of overweight people. See things through their eyes. In this way, you may be able to better anticipate their needs and concerns.

The chapters in this book were designed to address psychological and social issues common for the weight loss patient. Each chapter generally uses a problem solving approach, first articulating the issue and then providing suggestions for its amelioration. Although the sequence of chapters was designed be read in order, individual chapters may be read separately, either as a point of reference or to review previously learned information.

The information in the book hopefully will provide you with a better appreciation for the struggles faced by anyone who is overweight, as well as the challenges of those who contemplate and complete weight loss surgery. For many of these folks, surgery is only the beginning. Many find that losing weight after surgery is actually easier than making the behavioral and emotional changes that the surgery invokes. For this reason, the period after surgery marked by dramatic behavioral and emotional changes is when your role as a caregiver or professional is most crucial.

You've done your loved ones or patients a great service by picking up this book and volunteering to be of greater help to them. Thank you for your support!

Prologue: Life of the Fat Kid

WHAT DO I REMEMBER FROM childhood? If you've been wondering about my personal experience with weight, here's a glimpse.

On the Playground

It was another beautiful October day: fourth grade lunchtime recess in the schoolyard. My daily torment was about to commence. Dodgeball was truly hell on earth—the twentieth century's equivalent of thumbscrews or being drawn and quartered. But it didn't just destroy my body. It also devastated my mind and spirit.

The torture began immediately with the choosing of teams. I watched the two captains closely. The initial player selections were made quickly and decisively. Of course the jocks and the popular kids were first to be picked. The pace gradually slowed as the best of the best had been selected, with the remaining player selections requiring greater contemplation. As our numbers dwindled, eye contact with each other was avoided like the plague. The few of us that remained never spoke to one another and certainly not to the captains. I could never tell if the captains didn't look me in the eye because they were cowards or that they just pitied me. Finally, there were two of us left and I wondered how the final selection would be made—geek or fat kid? I prayed to the dodgeball gods, but knew it was pointless. It always turned out the same: Geek won, and I'm the last kid picked. Story of my life.

There I am, writhing in pain and the game itself has yet to begin. In truth, the pain of getting hit by a hard rubber ball traveling 40 miles an hour is *nothing* compared to the humiliation of the selection process that preceded it. The game itself was nothing more than a formality. The outcome really isn't much in question. But of course it wouldn't be bad enough to just be emotionally crippled by being the last of 22 children to be chosen, but now I'm about to get physically battered, as well. Who thought of this delightful sport? Clearly it wasn't a fat kid. The only good news is that the entire affair rarely lasted for more than a few rounds, at least for me.

There was always a lot of laughter on the playground. I could never tell if the other kids were laughing because they truly enjoyed the game, or were delighting in watching the lame fall. It's a bit chilling to think that one child might rejoice in providing another child with a circular welt that lasted for several weeks, but the jocks and the popular kids were often merciless. Kids being kids, I guess. I can remember the teachers prompting me to get off the back line and move up to try to pick up a loose ball or try to catch one. Sure, I'll go taunt the group of angry bulls with my new oversized red shorts and extra large yellow T-shirt. Every once in a while in a rage, I would get the guts to scoop up the ball and make a mad dash for center court, with the idea of exacting revenge on another poor soul, preferably the captain who opted not to pick me. But the story never played out with Goliath falling. In my story, David was fat and asthmatic. I tried desperately to hug the fence at the back of the court, but of course I always got nailed within two minutes. It's not hard to hit an elephant with a fastball from 20 feet away.

I can still vividly recall those moments and others like them. I hated gym class. How many times did I pretend to be sick to go to the nurse's office, just to avoid having to undress? And then there were those ridiculous state-mandated tests of physical fitness that we all had to take. They'd asked me to do five chin-ups. Then, I had to

climb a rope from the floor of the gym 30 feet up to the ceiling—
yeah, sure! The salamis hanging in my local deli would have a better
chance of climbing three inches up to the ceiling than I did climbing
those ropes.

Shopping for Clothes

Shopping for clothes was another delight. Each summer, my
mother would drag me through the husky boys' section of two awful department stores right before Labor Day. I would starve myself
the day before, praying the snaps on the pants would close, just this
once. And where did the term "husky" come from? To this day I still
don't understand what the relationship is between a beautiful white
snow dog and clothing for fat boys. It's actually quite ridiculous if
you think about it. Huskies valiantly dash through miles of snow.
I wheezed after walking the few steps to that hidden corner of the
husky boys' department, past the slim-cut Levi's that so many of my
classmates wore.

Oh yes, that was an additional treat. It wasn't bad enough that I
was eleven years old and 150 pounds, shopping for clothes in plain
sight of many of my thin, athletic classmates. I then had to spend
the next two hours accompanying my mother while she shopped for
bras and underwear. Somebody please shoot me!

"Husky" miraculously becomes "big and tall" when you reach
eighteen. What marketing geniuses abound in the clothing industry!
For women the language is truly confusing, and not knowing wom-
en's categories can be downright dangerous for us men. I remember
once asking my wife why she was shopping in the "petite" section,
given that she's 5'6" tall. I suggested she shop in the "woman" section because, after all, she *is* a woman. As you female readers might
imagine, this did not go well for me. I wasn't aware that "woman"
was the fashionista code word for "plus-sized" women. If there must
be a "plus-sized" department, shouldn't we call the section for super
thin women "minus-sized?" It's all *way* too confusing.

That Was Then...

High school was not an improvement for me. Dating was never a
problem. Then again, how can something you *don't* do be a problem?

I rarely attempted to even talk to girls until later in high school. Two hundred fourteen pound fifteen-year-olds rarely made the cover of "Tiger Beat." In fact, the only pain that lasted longer than the welt incurred during a game of dodgeball was the bruise my ego incurred after being teased by a gaggle of teenage girls as they strolled by my locker. There were a few girls who were my friends, and most of them were in the same boat as me. They weren't really any more interested in me than I was in them, but it was better than having no contact at all with the opposite sex. Collectively, our group was from the land of misfit toys. The geek, the fatty, the new kid, the brainiac, and more—our own version of "The Breakfast Club." But I was the fat kid, too deplorable for the actual movie. I thought about the pretty girls, but I don't think the favor was ever returned. Of course, in classic fashion, I was the friend of many attractive girls. I was the "nice guy" they were all willing to talk to, but nothing more. For those of you who are not aware, being called a nice guy as a teenage male is the kiss of death. Nice guys spend their weekends with mom and dad, not teenage girls.

Oh, I almost forgot! The absolute, indisputable, crème de la crème of humiliation occurred many years earlier. A torturous ritual so exquisite and inhumane, it's amazing that the Board of Education thought of it: The almost surreal experience of being lined up in weight order by the school nurse as a kindergartner. I could understand alphabetical order, but what could *possibly* be the purpose of lining up children by order of their weight? Perhaps, this was a ploy by the school board to humiliate me into dieting. Instead, it contributed to my desire to skip school, which I did with great regularity. I had lots of headaches and tummy aches that really weren't headaches and tummy aches at all. How could that be? My own school district shaming me into truancy? Indeed, they did.

As a kid, I frequently experienced two seemingly disparate feelings, often simultaneously, throughout my days at school. On some days, I would walk the hallways feeling like a 200-pound piñata. Everyone had a stick, and swinging at me was almost irresistible. I heard comments, got called all kinds of names, was teased, and generally felt like an outsider. Being fat made me very visible and quite unacceptable.

However, on other days, I felt almost completely invisible. Few said hello to me, many avoided eye contact, and smiles were doled out at a minimum. It was as if I wasn't even there. No one noticed me unless no one else was around. I felt alive during one-on-one interactions with my peers, but was an immediate casualty when a group began to form. When alone, people would talk to me; in a group, I was the invisible man. The experience of feeling both of these states—flickering on and off like a broken television—is almost surreal and quite uncomfortable. I was noticed by all of the mean kids whom I wished wouldn't notice me, and was all but ignored by the more popular kids with whom I wanted to develop friendships. It was the worst of both worlds.

Thankfully, the torment subsided by the latter high school years and college. By the end of high school, I was increasingly comfortable with the misfit gang and began not to care about those outside of our merry little band. At least that's what I wanted to believe. But with college looming, our group was about to split up and my emotional deck was about to get reshuffled. However, I tried to be positive by thinking that college could be great. Everyone gets a second chance and a clean slate, right? Everyone becomes the new kid, right? Wrong. My weight remained an issue. I entered the University of Florida at 5'9", weighing 214 pounds. I'm was in the land of bikinis and Speedos, wanting to wear a sweater covered by a parka. What was I *thinking*?

A small saving grace was a girlfriend I managed to meet at the end of high school. And while away at college, I made a few new friends. Maybe this time it would be different? No. My high school girlfriend of several years lost a significant amount of weight, and promptly dumped me for another guy.

I saw red. Enough was enough. I went on my first crazy restrictive diet and exercised like a madman. I dropped over 40 pounds within a few months. For the first time in my life, I was thin. Not thinner—*thin*. I fit into things I couldn't wear when I was twelve. I looked pretty good. I bought those expensive jeans and actually was able to fit into some shirts labeled "medium." I knew I wasn't an "extra large" anymore but I wasn't even a "large!" I don't think I could ever recall being a "medium!"

People responded to me differently, but I didn't feel much different inside. I remained a clown, with the seemingly extroverted, happy-go-lucky personality. The internal perception of who I was and how I thought others viewed me had crystallized over all those childhood years, and wasn't about to melt away with the loss of weight. And it showed: I was unassertive and nervous around others, especially girls. I felt awkward. I lost all of that weight and physically transformed into a new body. I finally looked like the person I always wanted to be. Only I kept the old brain. Thin body—fat brain. I desperately wanted it all to be in the past, but it wasn't. It turns out that the elementary school playground was the oven where my emotional cookies were baked. And at 21, weighing a mere 147 pounds, I still felt like a pile of crumbs.

...This Is Now

As I write these pages, I'm 175 pounds and without question I am in the best shape of my life. I exercise about four to five times each week in an established schedule. I monitor my daily caloric intake and lift weights several times a week. I'm compulsive about ensuring I keep my food and exercise routine.

I've lost more than 30 pounds three times in my life; and twice I gained it all back, with interest. I'd like to think that the third time was the charm, but I remain skeptical, very skeptical. As anyone who's ever lost a significant amount of weight knows, the weight is *begging* to return. If genetics, biology, and appetite are unrelenting, I must be, as well. I am determined to struggle and work hard to resist the return of those 30 pounds. And if the exercise and calorie monitoring keep those 30 pounds at bay, then I am blessed. Others have diseases that require far more invasive treatments.

Even with my weight loss accomplishment, those same old fat brain feelings occasionally sneak up on me. I still have a sense of somehow being unaccepted, like an outsider that needs to win people over to compensate for the fact that I'm fat, even though I'm not fat anymore. The irony is that some people go so far as to tell me that I'm thin. Thin? Thinner, maybe, but *thin*? What could be worse than being thin but feeling fat? The fat body is gone from my home, but I still hear those footsteps of fat brain creeping around in my attic.

Every once in a while, I still have feelings that I will be the last kid to be picked.

Childhood and adolescent experiences have a profound impact on the development of personality—of who you are, and who you will become. For me, I've accepted that my weight had a lot to do with the development of my sense of humor. Keep them laughing *with* you rather than *at* you. It's probably also why it has always been difficult for me to be assertive. In dodgeball, you learn to hug the back wall and avoid attention, lest you become too visible and get hit. Speaking up, being assertive, and trying to gain acceptance on my own merits is the equivalent of running to the centerline to grab the ball—suicide!

My struggle with my weight is similar to that of most people, considering the obesity epidemic that's spreading around the world. The media bombards us with studies about how fat we're all becoming and how gloomy the prospects are for us and our children, sitting around playing video games, chomping on potato chips, and drinking gallons of cola. It's going to take a lot of work to change our ways. And this is for the majority of us, who are only 10 to 30 pounds overweight.

But for those of us who need to lose 50, 75, or 100 pounds or more, the task of losing that much weight is monumental, seemingly impossible. Diet and exercise are frequently not enough. I often consider what I go through each day to keep my weight off, and the emotional struggle I've endured to fit in and make my way. But when I compare it to the struggle my patients have had, I am humbled. I have sat with hundreds of people whose lives have been decimated by weight. Many of my patients have told me that they feel like Swiss cheese, with so many holes poked in their lives. They describe the difficulty they have performing activities that most people take for granted, like putting on their shoes or climbing stairs. They reflect on so many of the wonders of life that they've had to let pass by.

Worst of all is the feeling of shame so many feel, faced with the rolling eyes and snickering stares from others, along with the seemingly acceptable discrimination that morbidly obese people experience almost every day. The public perception of obese people is appalling. They are viewed as lazy, stupid, unmotivated, and labeled with other demeaning attributes that are unfounded. In fact, in their constant struggle to lose weight and keep it off, no one works harder to accomplish a goal than most obese people do.

In the clinical literature, these negative perceptions of the obese have been demonstrated in study after study. And in my clinical practice, my patients recount story after story about the obtuse comments others make to them. They are extremely demoralized by the general public's view that their weight problem would be solved if they would just eat a little less and walk a little more, as if they haven't given the matter some thought and tried just about everything. As if!

My personal battles with my own weight have been extremely helpful when I work with those struggling with their weight. Many patients have recounted nightmares about their experiences with medical and other professionals regarding their weight. Insulting remarks, ridiculous diets, and the never-ending advice to diet and exercise, as if this is novel advice for anyone with a weight problem. As if.

"Gee doc, that's great advice! You mean I should eat less and move around some more? That's brilliant! I never thought of that! You're a genius!" So many of these well-meaning people just don't get it. It's time that everyone had a better grasp of the evidence, reality and truth about obesity, and the nightmare of losing weight. Read on.

Part I

Why Surgery?

As you contemplate your options for losing weight, one question you're sure to ask is why you should consider weight loss surgery. This section is designed to help you understand obesity, explore what weight loss surgery is all about, dispel myths about surgery, and set reasonable expectations for the aftermath of surgery. It reviews some of the barriers that make it so hard to lose weight, such as evolution, diets, and social stigma. Finally this section covers the fundamental knowledge necessary to help you make an informed decision about whether surgery is the right choice for you.

1

What Is Weight Loss Surgery?

S URGERY FOR WEIGHT LOSS IS a relatively new concept. Also known as bariatric surgery from the Greek *baros* meaning weight, weight loss surgery has been around for a little over 25 years. Although the first bariatric surgery was performed in 1954, the routine practice of weight loss surgery didn't hit its stride until the 1980's. In its early years, the surgery was generally reserved for people who were super morbidly obese, such as those weighing over 500 pounds, because the procedures were largely experimental and involved significant risk. Many of these early patients had considerable medical problems and had such profound impairment in their functioning that they had little to lose by trying surgery.

Today there are actually several different types of weight loss surgery. Over the past ten years, gastric bypass surgery has become the most popular type performed in the United States. More recently, gastric banding and gastric sleeve surgery, as well as other procedures have gained in popularity. There are differences between the various types of weight loss surgeries, both in terms of the procedures themselves as well as the medical and behavioral changes required to ensure long-term success. But their objective of providing lasting weight loss is the same. Weight loss surgery is now commonly performed laparoscopically, which is minimally invasive making surgery easier to accomplish and with fewer risks and complications. Determining which surgery is best for you depends on a number of complex factors, and this is an important discussion to have with your surgeon.

The number of hospitals offering weight loss surgery and surgeons performing them has increased considerably. The American Society for Metabolic and Bariatric Surgery (ASMBS) estimated that over 200,000 weight loss surgeries were performed in the United States in 2009, and that number is expected to increase. Bariatric surgery success stories are appearing in the popular media on a routine basis with a growing number of celebrities undergoing the procedures. Al Roker, the nationally known meteorologist, Carnie Wilson, performing artist with the Wilson Phillips group, and Khaliah Ali, daughter of Muhammad Ali, are among the growing list of big names who have had weight loss surgery.

Why So Popular?

Weight loss surgery is becoming more popular for a number of reasons. In many respects its growing popularity is the result of a shift in supply and demand. There has been a staggering increase in the number of morbidly obese people in the United States and throughout the world over the past 20 years, creating an ever-increasing supply of candidates for surgery. As weight loss surgeries become safer and insurance companies are more willing to pay, the demand for these procedures is increasing. As a result, the number of surgical weight loss programs is growing, with more and more hospitals offering surgery for weight loss.

Another reason for the increased popularity of surgical weight loss is that people are becoming more informed about the severe health consequences of morbid obesity. This is happening much in the same way as they became aware of the health consequences of cigarette smoking during the 1980's and 1990's. Consequences of obesity include Type II Diabetes, hypertension, elevated blood lipids, sleep apnea and other major medical problems. In general, the medical complications of morbid obesity diminish an individual's quality of life and shorten life span by a number of years. Physicians and patients alike are recognizing the urgency of treating morbid obesity.

The stigma of having weight loss surgery is declining, in turn fueling the growing popularity of surgery. More and more celebrities are making it known that they have had weight loss surgery, lighting the path for others to consider it. Additionally, as more magazines, Web sites and other media sources cover weight loss surgery, patients are able to learn about the surgery directly from those who have had it. And the news is generally positive.

The Biggest Reason

The biggest reason for the phenomenal growth of weight loss surgery is *because weight loss surgery works where little else does*. The clinical and scientific literature of treatments for morbid obesity tells us that surgery is the *only* treatment that truly works for most patients. Many of the best minds in medicine, psychology and behavior change will now concede this finding.

The reality is stark but true: Very few people lose 100 pounds through diet and exercise or currently available medications, and even fewer are able to keep the weight off for more than a few months. Individual testimonials and late night television miracle products aside, weight loss surgery is presently the only clinically established, long-term effective treatment for morbid obesity.

Through Thick and Thin

Now that you have a basic understanding of weight loss surgery and its growing popularity, your next question to me might be, "Okay doc, where do I sign up?" Not so fast. As I imply in the title of this book, weight loss surgery, along with everything that comes before and after it, is a journey. And this journey, like any other, has its rewards and its challenges.

Before we begin this journey, it's important to understand that the reasons we *gain* weight are distinct from the reasons we struggle to *lose* weight. I will address these separately, with chapter 2 focusing on weight gain, and chapters 3, 4, and 5 discussing barriers that stand in the way of weight loss. By exploring the dynamics of gaining and losing weight, you will have a better knowledge of how your body works to prepare you for chapter 6, which examines the most common questions about being a candidate for weight loss surgery.

Contrary to what you might think, this journey does not end once you're wheeled out of the operating room. The remainder of the book, starting with chapter 7, will help you navigate the challenges of life after surgery. You'll learn to deal in a new way with hunger, emotional eating, slips, and relapse. You'll also be introduced to tools that will help you deal with the new you, both in terms of your own reaction to life after surgery as well as the reaction of others around you.

This book was designed to be your road map throughout your weight loss journey, to help you understand where you've been, to clarify where you're going, and to anticipate what things will be like along the way. It is my hope that this book will bring many issues regarding weight loss into better perspective. Ultimately, I trust you'll be able to make an informed and sound decision about whether weight loss surgery is the right choice for you.

2

What Is Obesity?

A GOOD PLACE TO START this journey is to gain a better understanding of obesity and its causes. Weight loss surgery is a solution to a major problem, and that problem is morbid obesity.

Obesity 101

Let's clarify some of the medical jargon used with regard to weight. The term *overweight* simply means that you weigh more than the American Medical Association's recommended guidelines say you should weigh. Currently, I weigh 175 pounds. According to my doctor, given my height of 5'8", I should weigh between 155 and 160 pounds. Clinically speaking, I am 15 to 20 pounds overweight. It is estimated that more than 50 percent of American adults are overweight by this definition. Most Americans are in the same boat, and it's sinking fast!

A healthy weight for one person might be quite unhealthy for another, and much is dependent on height. It is for this reason we sometimes use the body mass index (BMI), which is a statistical measure of body size based on both weight and height. To calculate your

BMI, multiply your weight in pounds by 703, and divide that product by your height, in inches squared. For example, for my current weight of 175 pounds and height of 5'8" (68 inches), my BMI is:

$$(175 \text{ pounds} \times 703) \div (68 \text{ inches})^2 = 26.6$$

The term *obese* means that you weigh 20 percent more than the recommended guidelines say you should weigh, or that your BMI is between 30 and 40. So when I weighed 214 pounds in high school, I was considered obese. Most people who believe they're only slightly overweight are alarmed to discover that they are in fact obese. Consider that if I weighed 190, I would be obese according to the 20 percent guideline. If I weighed 198, I would be obese according to the BMI guideline. These are not difficult lines to cross.

The next step is *morbid obesity*. Being morbidly obese means that you weigh 100 pounds more than the recommended guidelines, or that your BMI is 40 or higher. If my bathroom scale ever reaches 255 pounds, I would be morbidly obese according to the 20 percent guideline. If that scale breaches 264, the BMI guideline would signal morbid obesity.

As you can see, morbid obesity is different from obesity, and much different from being overweight. At first glance it may appear that morbid obesity is simply a more severe version of obesity, but this is not the case. The body of a morbidly obese person does not function in the same way as the body of someone who is 25 pounds overweight. It also does not respond to obesity treatments as someone who needs to lose 25 pounds.

The original target audience for weight loss surgery was almost exclusively patients with morbid obesity. Most of today's weight loss surgery patients are indeed morbidly obese. However, recent research suggests that individuals who have a BMI from 35 to 40 and have other problems related to their weight also may benefit from weight loss surgery. More and more folks in this category are currently receiving the surgery.

The Disease of Obesity

In recent years, the medical community has designated obesity as a *disease*. Morbid obesity is a more complex and severe form of the disease. With this designation, there will be a dramatic change in the way we view and address morbid obesity.

What is a disease? Commonly used definitions suggest that there needs to be some impairment of health or some type of abnormal functioning to qualify as a disease. Defined in this way, obesity is clearly a disease, because we know that obesity both impairs health and causes abnormal functioning. This is even more so for those with morbid obesity.

Although not without some controversy, mounting scientific evidence and medical consensus have accepted the definition of obesity as a disease. Heading the evidence list is the genetic tendency toward obesity, which is both metabolic and behavioral. In other words, obesity occurs mostly because of disturbances in the body's regulation of fat and calories, but also because of biologically based abnormalities in food cravings, satiety (feeling full) and eating patterns.

There are some who are skeptical about the designation of obesity as a disease, and these skeptics usually point to one or more of the following reasons:

1. An individual's behavior, such as eating and inactivity, is essential to the cause of obesity.

2. The human gene pool hasn't changed sufficiently in the past 20 years to cause the recent large increase in the prevalence of obesity.

3. Not all obese people are unhealthy.

4. The "disease" designation could inhibit efforts to help people take responsibility for their weight.

These four criticisms do hold some validity. However, the first three discount obesity as a disease because critics are taking the view that a disease is either solely genetic or not. Obesity is clearly a combination of genetic, biological and behavioral influences. It appears that genetics provide the "seeds" for obesity while environment and behavior supply the "water" that makes it flower. In fact, most diseases today, including heart disease, cancer, stroke and AIDS, are partly, if not significantly, determined by lifestyle and behavioral choices. Obesity is the end result of poor lifestyle and genetics in the same way that lung cancer or heart attacks can be the end result of cigarette smoking and genetics. Plus, there's growing evidence that all obese people are at higher risk of premature death. This is similar to people who have elevated cholesterol levels, which clearly has been declared a medical condition worthy of professional care.

The fourth criticism seems unlikely because people will always want to lose weight, and calling obesity a disease would unlikely diminish that desire. In fact, the opposite could occur: People may begin to acknowledge obesity as a condition that is dangerous requiring serious attention, rather than something merely annoying or unsightly. With the designation of obesity as a disease, people may very well take their responsibility to address their weight more seriously.

The Stigma Still Exists

This shift to viewing obesity as a disease is far from complete, as many of my patients can attest when their physician or family made efforts to intervene regarding their weight. Many report that their doctors didn't make any suggestions beyond cursory advice to eat less and exercise. Occasionally they would be given a prescription for the latest weight loss drug. Others indicated that their doctors made a few suggestions like cutting down on carbohydrates or joining a gym.

When I was tipping the scale close to 200 pounds, I recall my doctor giving me a photocopied page of a very calorie-restrictive diet, recommending that I eat no more than 800 calories a day. He told me that I should start exercising, but had no suggestions as to what exercises or how often to do them. He told me that my weight was unhealthy. He didn't ask any questions about my dietary habits or the effect the weight was having on my quality of life. He even belittled the problem by joking about it!

I felt confused and overwhelmed by my weight. I also felt ashamed and embarrassed for being so heavy. I never went back to that doctor. Countless patients tell me that my experience was not unlike their experience with their own doctors, many of whom also never went back. Although such practices certainly do not characterize all doctors, when they do occur in can be humiliating if not devastating.

My patients tell me that their families are often just as harsh. Sometimes there is name-calling or efforts to restrict food, hide food, or some other drastic measure. These tactics generally make the morbidly obese person feel ashamed, embarrassed, and stupid. Not surprisingly, other negative emotions can also creep in, such as anxiety and depression. Such approaches do not generally "rally the troops" and they rarely lead to sustained weight loss. In fact, they often lead to feelings of hopelessness, more eating and more weight gain.

A Shift in Perspective

As more and more health providers, family and friends begin to adopt the concept of morbid obesity as a disease, we can start thinking of it as a chronic and complicated phenomenon requiring a well-developed solution, rather than a simple and temporary problem that is resolved with simple advice. By designating morbid obesity as a disease, two enormous changes would come about:

1. Morbid obesity would be viewed as a significantly more complicated and formidable problem that is not easily resolved with remedies such as diet and exercise.

2. We would stop blaming patients for having the condition, instead providing empathy and support to explore healthy solutions. If we are the patients, we would stop blaming and deprecating ourselves, as well.

Consider how other diseases are addressed and treated compared to what typically happens with morbid obesity. When a physician believes that a patient may have a disease like congestive heart failure, a number of tests are conducted, referrals are made and treatment options are explored. It is as if an alarm has been sounded and a call to action has been made. A good physician is very much involved in this process, providing information, reassurance and support and making herself available to the patient as needed. The doctor is generally not judgmental of the patient for having the disease.

Similarly, most family members are supportive when they learn that their loved one has a disease. Support and encouragement are offered. A caring family rallies together and does whatever is necessary to care for the afflicted loved one. The patient doesn't blame himself for the condition and doesn't become overwhelmed with guilt and shame for having the disease. When a disease is defined, treatment is sought, action is taken, and support and encouragement are provided. This is what we need for obesity.

The Causes of Obesity

Obesity and morbid obesity are diseases that are partly defined as weighing too much. Obvious questions to ask include: How did I gain all this weight? Why did I gain all this weight? Why do some people gain so much weight while others do not? The answers require us to take a closer look at the causes of obesity.

Sometimes the answer is straightforward: Obese people eat too much! Other times it's less obvious. Case in point: We all know people who seem to eat as much or even more than we do, yet they've never had a weight problem. Therefore, ingesting too many calories is almost always part of the story, but rarely the whole story.

It seems reasonable to hold yourself accountable for having gained weight; after all, you're the one who chose to put the Devil Dogs in your mouth right? Don't we have free choice?

Well, yes and no.

Genetics, hormones, medications, your culture, emotional reasons and other factors play an enormous role in motivating us to eat and to gain weight. As you will soon see, the Devil Dog almost puts itself into your hand. Some of these factors we can change and others, we cannot. Let's take a closer look at some of the influences on weight gain.

Genetics

Genetics may be the granddaddy of all causes, given the power of heredity. Studies of twins indicate that about 50 to 70 percent of the tendency toward obesity is inherited. Similarly, studies show that when both parents are obese, the chance their children also will be obese is 60 to 80 percent. In contrast, when both parents are thin, the likelihood of a child becoming obese is only about nine percent.

Of course the home environment might account for these differences in the weight of children. It is for this reason researchers turn to adoption studies to understand the differential emphasis of genetics and environment. In some of the best adoption studies, when adopted children are reared apart from biological parents, it turns out that there is a strong relationship between the BMI of adoptees and their biological parents, but a very weak if any relationship between the BMI of adoptees and their adoptive parents. Such findings point to the strong influence of genetic factors on body size.

The upshot is that obesity runs in families. So it isn't just Aunt Francesca's amazing lasagna. If you are morbidly obese, it is very likely that some of your siblings or parents are obese or morbidly obese, as well. As one woman jokingly said to me, "It's because of my genes that I can't fit into my jeans!"

We do not know much about the specific genetics of obesity in humans, but we do know that obesity is, in part, an inherited trait. So even before you swallowed that first spoonful of strained peas, you already had one strike against you.

Hormones and Metabolism

Recently, the impact of hormones has been receiving tremendous attention in the clinical and scientific literatures. Two hormones in particular, ghrelin and leptin frequently appear in newspaper headlines citing research about the potential causes of obesity.

Ghrelin is a hormone that has been implicated in the stimulation of hunger. Ghrelin levels increase before meals and decrease after meals. Leptin induces satiation when present at higher levels. Put simply, the release of ghrelin contributes to creating hunger, thus stimulating us to eat. The release of leptin seems to be involved in the feelings of satiety, and so contributes to our sensation that it is time to stop eating.

We also know that metabolism plays a role in the cause of obesity as well as in our difficulty with losing weight. For example, because our metabolism changes with age, most of us will gradually gain some weight as we age. This may also explain why it is harder to lose weight and keep it off as we get older.

Medication

Several medications are known to increase weight such as steroids and antidepressants. I have treated a number of patients who have gained over 25 pounds within a year of initiating such medications. Ask anyone who has been on an anti-inflammatory drug for several months and you will hear about the anxiety they experienced regarding seemingly out of control weight gain.

Those with Type II Diabetes often face a similar problem. This type of diabetes is often caused, in part, by excessive body weight. But unfortunately many of the medications used to *treat* this diabetes actually *contribute* to weight gain, leading to a truly vicious cycle!

Activity Level

There are two types of activity. The first is the general level of necessary activity that we get each day by going about the usual business of living life. The second is the amount of activity we elect to do in addition to what is necessary. The latter is what we call exercise.

Our technological "progress" has greatly diminished the need for daily activity. Many of us work in professions that require us to do little more than sit for hours upon hours while typing and clicking on a computer. Worse yet, an increasing number of us spend an additional one to four hours sitting in a train or car commuting to and from our sedentary job. For many, the walk to and from the car and to and from the bathroom is all the activity we do during the day.

Technology has dramatically cut down on the calories required to perform household chores, much of which can be completed simply by pushing buttons or turning dials. Washing clothes, cleaning dishes, cooking food, shopping, communicating and many of our occupations can be performed with very little activity.

For these reasons and others, adding exercise to our activity roster has become necessary. Fifty years ago, adding exercise to our daily routines was less common and less necessary as people received plenty of activity simply by doing what needed to be done every day.

Washing clothes, walking to stores, cleaning the house and many jobs were significantly more physically demanding and burned lots of calories. Now, we have to go out of our way to exercise and it can be quite difficult to keep it going. As our lives become busier, it's challenging to find the time and the will to exercise. It's difficult to consistently wake up at 5 A.M. to exercise before work, or to exercise at 8 P.M. after having spent eight or more hours working and another two hours commuting to and from work.

Quite a few of my patients can recall past success in keeping weight off through a rigorous program of diet and daily exercise. Some also recall that once they were physically injured and couldn't run five miles every morning anymore, or once their job schedule changed, the whole program started to crumble. It's not that exercise cannot help us lose weight. Rather it's the amount we need and the consistency with which we need it that is daunting. And most of us have a problem keeping it going for one reason or another.

Exercise can also problematically be restricted by cultural factors. As our American lifestyle is viewed as desirable and spreads throughout the world, so have some elements of our sedentary routine. As a result, obesity is now becoming an epidemic in areas where it was rarely seen before, such as the Far East. What may have begun as an American phenomenon is no longer confined to our borders.

Culture

Whether it is your nationality or religious tradition, cultural factors have a profound influence on eating behavior and food choices. Human evolution has made us predisposed to be very interested in seeking out food and wanting to eat. Our evolutionary imperative for survival essentially screams, "Get food!" And our individual culture influences what foods we get and when to eat them.

Whether you're Italian, Irish, French, Mexican, Cuban, Chinese, Jewish or from any other group, there are specific foods and eating traditions related to your particular culture. When you consider almost any major life event, it is completely intertwined with food and eating—weddings, engagements, bar mitzvahs, baptisms, confirmations, births, birthdays, anniversaries—yum, yum, yum!

Holidays are all about food. It doesn't matter what group you

identify with. You name the holiday and there are special foods associated with it. In fact, food is often the primary focus of the holiday.
For example, Thanksgiving seems more about binging on turkey and
all the trimmings than about giving thanks, except for perhaps a
brief bit of formal gratitude for all that food lying before us.

In the United States, we have taken the behavior of eating to an
entirely higher level. We invented an enormous fast food and snack
industry that spends millions of dollars each year encouraging us to
eat high-calorie high-fat unhealthy food using well-researched marketing and advertising gimmicks such as supersizing, buy one get one
free, and other cute tricks. Food has become cheap, quick, and easy
to acquire.

Too many Americans eat high-calorie fast food and high-calorie snacks on a regular basis. Yes, it is true that individuals have
the ability to make food choices for themselves. And fast foods and
snacks are just one available choice. But our innate urge to eat and
to respond to food cues, along with an increasingly busy lifestyle and
readily available fast foods and snacks, are a nightmarish combination. This problem is no longer confined to the United States, as lives
have become busier and as fast food chains and processed snacks
gradually have become prevalent worldwide.

For some of us, the workplace has become a gluttonous environment, as well. Many business meetings occur with food. Go into the
boardroom of any major corporation and in the middle of the big,
brown, mahogany table sit several platters or baskets of food that we
probably shouldn't be eating. Food is also a popular business gift.

Social gatherings commonly involve food. Dinner and a movie is
perhaps the single most popular weekend activity for most folks. And
what would a movie be without a two-gallon tub of popcorn?! If the
gathering is to be at someone's home, most of us are taught to bring
something to eat or a beverage to drink. Feeding people is seen as an
expression of endearment.

I know what you're going to say: "But doc, couldn't you make
healthy choices instead of ordering tons of Chinese food? Couldn't
you simply have one or two pigs in a blanket at the wedding rather than 17? Couldn't you just have a small serving of turkey and
mashed potatoes on Thanksgiving? Couldn't you have stopped at

one piece of pie instead of three?" My answer would be: "Certainly, but our human 'hard wiring' combined with this increasingly challenging environment in which we live makes it very difficult to just say no." And even those folks who do successfully resist at first are often unable to do so for very long.

Emotional Factors

Sure, I eat a little more when I'm down in the dumps. It makes me feel better. Ever eat an Oreo that didn't make you feel better for at least a few seconds? And if you eat 30 of them, that's a comfy half hour! It's hard to just say no. Of course, while you were medicating your feelings with food, those additional calories were busily contributing to your waistline.

Emotional eating is very much related to weight gain because of the types of foods we eat. I've never met a patient who confesses to eating broccoli or celery when they are looking for an emotional pick-me-up. Sweets and comfort foods usually rule the day.

The link between emotions and eating is very complex. Although emotional eating is partly a learned behavior, there is likely a biological basis for our tendency to eat when in distress. We will frequently visit the interplay between emotions and eating throughout this book.

Gender

There are interesting anecdotal differences between men and women when it comes to food choices and eating behavior. It doesn't happen all the time, but in my experience women seem much more likely to go for the sweets when stress kicks in, whereas men generally will have a fourth meal or the like. Interestingly, even among the women who tell me they don't generally eat sweets, they often will during their menstrual cycle. Scientists may have not yet uncovered the reasons, but most women that I've met readily acknowledge that there is clear relationship between their cycle and their desire for chocolate.

Another interesting difference in the eating patterns of men and women is that women commonly report that they are more likely to graze throughout the day, whereas men generally will prefer to consume large meals. This may be the result of the social pressures our culture places on women. However, most women tell me that they will rarely eat two pieces of cake in a sitting, but rather pick at the cake throughout a day until half of it is gone. On the other hand, when men finally sit down to have some dessert, they will eat two or three pieces in one shot.

A growing body of research strongly suggests that women's bodies horde fat and don't let go of it relative to men's bodies. Also, men have a greater percentage of muscle mass as compared to women. These findings may explain why men lose weight faster than women, and why exercise seems to have a more significant impact on weight loss for men relative to women.

All of these varied gender differences likely occur due to a combination of genetics and environmental exposure, and I'm certain future research will help clarify the causes.

It's Not Just One Thing

Even if you haven't been paying complete attention to all these details, there is one thing I want you to take with you from this chapter: *It's not just one thing.* A multitude of factors influence eating and weight gain, and ultimately obesity. You can easily see that there is a lot more going on than that oft cited mantra of "calories in—calories out."

It also would be rather naïve to suggest that the factors I presented above tell the entire story. There are likely a number of other influences on eating and weight gain that we have yet to discover.

In the next chapter, I'll deal with the flip side of weight gain, namely weight loss. Why is it so hard to lose weight? Let's find out.

3

The Power of Evolution

S OME OF THE CHOICES WE make, both choices of environment and choices of behavior, influence obesity. Such choices may have prevented us from becoming overweight in the first place, and may help prevent future generations from becoming overweight, as well. If our next generations of children improve what they eat and adopt a more active lifestyle, their struggle with obesity will almost certainly be reduced.

Regarding such choices, here is one of the more important points I'm going to make in this book:

> Your choices and behavior *are* partly responsible for your obesity. However, your choices and behavior *are not* exclusively to blame for your inability to lose weight and keep it off.

Once an individual is obese, their struggle is largely predetermined. They are going to fight a never-ending uphill battle to lose the weight and keep it off. The human body's processes that relate to eating, appetite, satiety (feeling full) and weight regulation are extremely complex and not very well understood. What exactly makes us hungry? What makes us full? What makes us feel unsatisfied or want to keep eating even when we know we're physically full? We do not have clear answers to these questions.

At first glance, the method to lose weight appears quite simple: Consume fewer calories than you need and you will lose weight. Calories are actually units of energy, and in this model, food and the calories it contains are fuel. And your body needs this fuel to operate properly. Obesity in this model is an excess of stored fuel. Losing weight requires either taking in less fuel (fewer calories) than the body needs to operate over a sustained period of time, or burning up excess fuel through activity. Both of these methods would require the body to go into its fat stores to make up for the calorie deficit to continue to operate properly. As a consequence of this sustained need to go into the body's excess calorie storage, you would lose weight.

So there you have it: Good old diet and exercise are all you need to lose weight. In theory, the process sounds simple. In reality, unfortunately, the story is much more complicated.

A number of processes the body employs greatly complicate and thwart our efforts to lose weight. We become hungry. We become irritable and think incessantly about what to eat. We start to fantasize about food. At first glance, this all seems rather odd. Why is my body trying to stop me from losing weight when it would clearly benefit me to do so? Why is my body trying to hurt me? Evolution provides many of the answers.

Evolutionary Influences on Weight

Understanding how evolution impacts weight in human society requires us to turn back the clock more than 50,000 years or so. At that time most humans were hunter-gatherers, living in nomadic groups and wandering about without permanent settlements. Food was quite scarce. A group of hungry humans would venture out each morning and try to spear a gazelle or antelope for dinner. They'd be lucky if they caught one gazelle per week and would likely expend thousands of calories in the process. Trust me, if you've ever tried to hunt for a gazelle with a sharpened stick you'd understand completely! Maybe these early humans would be lucky enough to kill a rat or a few squirrels along the way when the gazelle hunt wasn't so successful. Insects were probably a significant source of protein, as well. Yum! (Don't cringe, but most cultures still consume insects as a major protein source.)

Although fruits and vegetables were always a significant part of human diets, we were primarily carnivores or meat eaters. Therefore, we were very reliant on hunting for food. Plants were not yet domesticated. There were no crops being cultivated. There were only a few wild fruits and vegetables around and these were only available during limited times of the year and only in certain locations. Fishing may have existed but probably wasn't much easier than hunting, considering that they used sticks and not fishing poles.

Early humans typically didn't live beyond their twenties or thirties and likely had a number of diseases related to malnutrition. If the human species were to survive, it would have to develop a system that would enable it to go very long periods of time with very little fuel, almost like a car that could travel 5,000 miles on one tank of gas. Scientists tell us that such a system is exactly what evolved. The human body was perfectly designed to go long distances and long periods of time with very little fuel. If this system had not evolved, humans would probably now be extinct. The human species scratched by on whatever sources of calories were available. Having an *excess* of calories was hardly a concern and neither was getting enough exercise. Ever try to spend your day chasing after gazelles? Even squirrels can give you a good workout. The prehistoric lifestyle involved expending tremendous amounts of calories to catch and kill precious few calories.

Basic agricultural practices began about 10,000 years ago, prompting the Neolithic Revolution when access to food surplus led to the formation of permanent human settlements, the domestication of animals, and the use of metal tools. Agriculture encouraged trade and cooperation between settlements, leading to the development of complex societies. However, the daily life of a typical human still required expending a tremendous number of calories while consuming precious few. In addition, humans were eating whole foods since no processing or additives were yet available. The norm was to eat moderate amounts of whole foods while engaging in a great amount of daily activity.

This magnificent human machine worked very well for a long time. Even well into the twentieth century, famines and food shortages were common, so this incredible human system that could operate on very little fuel remained adaptive and necessary. The human species proliferated across the globe.

However, during the past 50 years, not even a spec in the evolutionary timeline, a radical change has occurred. The human environment has changed dramatically and in ways that perfectly explain why the number on the bathroom scale is climbing.

Fast Forward to the Modern Era

Over the past few hundred years, food technology advanced remarkably, significantly improving how we grow crops and domesticate animals. Food availability has become more controllable and predictable. The industrial revolution and the advent of machines have dramatically advanced the technology of food production, and the computer age has made the advance even more rapid. These changes can be seen from changed farming practices to the synthesis of new foods, all at the expense of relying on what exists in nature.

Machines have allowed humans to plant crops on enormous tracts of land, irrigate the fields, and then pick the crops in record time and with precision. With irrigation technology, we are less dependent on the weather. Furthermore, we now enjoy a global economy so when we can't grow a crop during the winter in the United States we can import it from another region of the world.

Canning, preserving, refrigeration and other modern technologies have also improved food availability and now allow food to last for years! We live in the age of supermarkets. Only a few years ago, people went to a butcher for their meat, a produce store for their fruits and vegetables, and a bakery for their bread. Today it's one stop shopping in almost every town in America. Cooking has become an American pastime and cooking methods at home have improved, as well.

Growing food, acquiring food and preparing food have become much easier, but the environment that we designed over the course of thousands of years no longer exists. In the thousands of years of human existence, the past 50 years is the only time we have had to deal with the problem of excess food. Fifty years is a blink of an eye in the scope of human history. Ask your grandparents or great-grandparents that emigrated from Europe or elsewhere during the late 19th century or early 20th century, or who experienced the great depression in America, about the problem of having *too many* calories when they were children, and you'll get a good chuckle out of them.

No Time to Evolve

So here we are in the present with a surplus of food and calories all around us, stuck with a human body that has been perfectly tuned over thousands of years to operate on very few calories in a calorie-poor environment, while requiring lots and lots of activity and exercise merely to exist. As you by now have surmised, our current human body has not had enough time to evolve to our new calorie-rich environment. In fact, our body is perfectly designed for the exact *opposite* environment in which we now live!

Our highly evolved brains have figured out how to kill gazelles, pack them in cellophane, box them in ice, and ship them anywhere in the world directly to your door 365 days per year. Very few of us will ever need to fish, hunt or grow our own food. We now have calories on demand without the need to burn a single calorie to acquire them. For the first time in human history, we are running a calorie surplus.

And what does your nifty present-day human body do with all of those extra calories? Your body does the same with those extra calories as you do with the mongo-sized 100-count fun-sized value packs of cheesy curls that you bought in your local megastore: It puts them in the closet! Your body's closet is your hips, butt, thighs, and... You get the picture. Your body stocks up on all those extra calories you consume because it was designed to live in an environment as if it was 20,000 B.C., believing that it could be another month before you catch that next gazelle.

The problem, of course, is that you will catch your next gazelle in less than four hours. And what a gazelle it is! A 1,500-calorie bonanza at an all-you-can-eat Chinese buffet! Gradually, your body becomes your enemy. It's stuck on this idea of conserving extra fuel to better cope with the next famine. But the famine never comes, so the extra supply of fuel is never used and you're left dragging around that pantry of extra food in your XXXL jeans.

Now you have a better appreciation of the reasons why it is truly so difficult to lose weight and keep it off. You have thousands of years of human evolution that have made us into incredibly efficient machines, perfectly designed to get by on very few calories. Now add to that factors we discussed in the previous chapter, such as human genetics, hormones, metabolism, cultural experiences, and that toxic all-you-can-eat environment.

And what is your weapon of choice to fight back? That latest wonder diet from the magazine at the checkout counter at your supermarket? Good luck! Read on to discover why diets are probably not your best friend.

4

Why Diets Don't Work

MUCH OF THE DISCUSSION ABOUT our national obesity epidemic focuses on those of us who need to lose about 25 pounds or so. When you extend the discussion to those battling morbid obesity, the concept of dieting becomes almost ridiculous.

True, there are genuine problems with our eating habits and our increasingly sedentary lifestyle, where many of us do little more than push buttons all day long. And of course, you didn't become overweight completely by accident. Your behavior did have something to do with it. Some of those trips to the food court at the shopping mall didn't help. But as I hope I've convinced you by now, the problem of losing weight is far more complicated than that.

This is especially relevant when we are talking about morbid obesity where someone needs to lose 100 pounds or more. As you know from chapter 3, the human body is wonderfully tuned to get by on very few calories, but abysmal at getting rid of the excess fat that results from having ingested too many extra ones.

If the body has difficulty ridding itself of 10 to 20 pounds of extra calories, it must be close to impossible to remove 100 pounds worth, right? Exactly right! And how do most of us try to get rid of those extra calories? We engage in the activity that is perhaps one of the most hated words in the English language, the mother of all four-letter words: DIET.

Trying That New Diet

It's Monday morning and you decide to start that trendy diet you just read about in the magazine you were browsing at the checkout counter at the local megastore where you bought your 100-pack of snack-sized cheesy blasts. Maybe you're fortunate and you win the first few battles. You've lost seven pounds in the first ten days. Terrific! Now here comes a weekend barbecue. Man those burgers smell good and that potato salad looks mighty fine. I'll just have two tablespoons, you say to yourself. Whew, that was close.

Now it's week number three on the diet, and for some reason I've only lost two pounds this week. I knew it would slow down a bit; that's okay. There's catered lunch at work: Brownies, cookies, they all smell so good. I'll just have two small cookies. I've earned them. At the next weigh in, I notice I only lost one more pound. That's strange. I wonder what's going on. I also notice that I'm getting hungrier than I was two weeks ago. In fact, I'm walking around starving. And I'm thinking about food constantly. I'm planning my dinner just after I've eaten breakfast; that can't be normal.

Why can't I just eat like everyone else? Okay, that's the negative thinking my psychologist was talking about. I'll just think more rational thoughts instead. And I'll drink more water like everyone says I should. Well I know that if I'm going to beat this obesity thing, I won't be able to just "wing it." I've got to write things down and exercise more.

At the gym that night I walk for 30 minutes and I'm soaked with sweat. The calorie meter on my treadmill says I burned 125 calories. Good for me! Now, I'll shower up and have an energy bar as a treat. Yum, that was good; I wonder how many calories it has. Wow—350! Oh my God, that's almost three hours on the treadmill. Who has that kind of time? Okay, tomorrow I'll start doing 45 minutes.

Later in the week we celebrate Janet's birthday party in the office. They brought in Chinese food. Boy that was good. Of course I had a little General Tso's chicken, my favorite, and a fortune cookie. Oh yeah, Janet said I had to have a piece of her birthday cake. But, it was just a small piece. Unfortunately, I had to stay late at the office the past two nights so I couldn't get to the gym.

Next weigh in and I gained two pounds! What? I *gained* two pounds? This is unbelievable! I'm frustrated. I've been good nine out of ten days. I'm watching what I eat. In general, I'm living on salads and other rabbit food. My four-year-old eats more than I do! I'm exercising as much as I can possibly fit it into my schedule, and I've *gained* two pounds!

Sound familiar?

Diet Defined

You must know that it's not a good start when the word you are trying to define begins with the word "die!"

So, what is a diet exactly? A diet is a temporary intervention designed to address a chronic problem. Without really giving it much consideration, most of us go "on" a diet with every expectation that we will eventually go "off" the diet, yet we expect the results to endure. It's kind of silly if you think about it. We actually *believe* that the diet will "cure" the obesity. You take a headache medication expecting it to "cure" your headache and antacids to "cure" your heartburn. Generally, this works. The same cannot be said for dieting. It often doesn't even work in the short run much less the long run.

If a diet were to truly work, we would have to stay on it or at least a modified version of it forever. This immediately eliminates most of the diets out there. You can't live forever on chocolate powdered dust, or eat only grapefruits or steak and bacon for the next 40 years, at least not most people. In fact, many diets outwardly state that they are not to be used for more than a few weeks. So if you need to get into a particular dress by next Friday, maybe the asparagus soup diet is for you. If you're trying to lose weight and keep it off for the duration of your life, perhaps not.

From Diets to Lifestyle Changes to Reality

The diet industry is beginning to catch on and has shifted to using the phrase "lifestyle change" rather than diet. More and more diet programs are recommending and advertising a balanced, healthy diet focused primarily on portion control. The tag line "for life" is commonly in their advertisements. Yes, it's a welcome change and in theory, a reasonable concept: Stay on the diet for life and it will work. The problem is that most human beings can't stay on a major diet for the rest of their lives. We have major difficulty staying on a regimen for more than a month, let alone a lifetime! Perhaps behavioral science will figure it out someday, but at present it generally doesn't work.

It's all noble and well and good that the diet industry is promoting a complete lifestyle makeover. It sounds good and plays well in their ads. But I'll let you in on a little secret. Here's what the diet industry doesn't want you to know:

> Most interventions designed to help reduce a person's weight by more than 10 to 20 pounds are typically ineffective.

Hundreds of well-designed clinical weight loss studies at premier universities throughout the world have demonstrated that losing about 25 pounds through diet and exercise and keeping it off for more than a year is unlikely. Usually less than ten percent of those who attempt it will ever succeed.

To be clear, this statistic applies to those who need to lose 25 pounds and attempt to keep it off for more than a year. Less than ten percent can do it. Now, if you expand the research findings to folks who are morbidly obese and need to lose 100 or more pounds, the numbers of those who succeed shrink even further.

Now you understand why people who actually accomplish this feat are featured on the front of national magazines or on daytime talk shows. It's an improbable but amazing achievement! Imagine winning the lottery twice in the same year and you get the picture. Consider that what is possible is not the same as what is common. While it is theoretically *possible* to lose 100 pounds with diet alone, it is extremely *unlikely*. Is it possible to lose 100 pounds and keep it off for ten or more years? Yes. Is it likely? An emphatic no!

So why do we keep beating ourselves up for our inability to pull it off? If you think about it, condemning yourself for not being able to lose 100 pounds and keep it off is no different than condemning yourself for not being as intelligent as Albert Einstein. After all, you could study nine hours a day and learn quantum physics. It is theoretically possible, right? The logic that says that you could lose 100 pounds and keep it off for several years or more is the same logic that says you could become the next Albert Einstein. It's possible, but not likely. And I don't know a single person who feels guilty that they're not as smart as Einstein. But I know many who feel guilty over their failed attempts to lose weight.

The basic concept of a diet, even a lifestyle change, is simple enough and seems rational: Eat less and you will lose weight, whether you're 25 or 100 pounds overweight. But the best scientific research, the smartest doctors in the most prestigious of clinics, and the most honest real-world experience of so many who have tried it all know one very sobering bit of reality: It rarely works. So why do we keep riding the diet merry-go-round?

My Diet Conspiracy Theory

The blame should be placed on two doorsteps: (1) myths perpetuated by the diet industry, and (2) our collective ignorance. The latter is primarily a consequence of the former, as well as the foolish belief that what is possible for one person is probable for all persons. The diet industry has perpetuated the great myth that it is possible for most people to lose weight and keep it off for good.

"But Dr. Huberman, I know someone who has lost 63 pounds and kept it off for three years!"

"But Dr. Huberman, my cousin did it!"

"But Dr. Huberman, I keep seeing people on my favorite television talk show who have lost the weight!"

Of course there are a handful of folks who have been successful. I applaud those who have managed to accomplish significant long-term weight loss through diet and exercise; it's an incredible victory. But this is not the case for the majority of those who have ever attempted to lose weight through these methods. I realize that this is a controversial assertion and that it has ruined my chances for ever appearing in anyone's diet ad, so before you sharpen your nails for the attack, humor me and answer this question:

> How many people do you know that have lost 25 pounds
> through diet and exercise *and* have successfully kept it off
> for five years or more?

Got one or two? Good! Now compare that number to the total number of people that you know who have been unsuccessful at accomplishing this same feat. Don't forget to add up each time they tried, not just the number of people. The ratio is horrendous, isn't it? Most people know at least ten people who have lost and regained 10 to 20 pounds on several occasions, only to have it come back each time. Now imagine what those numbers would look like if you had a group of friends who needed to lose 100 pounds!

Here's another way to think about the problem. If any one of these commercial diets or advertised weight loss miracles actually worked for most folks, then why are there hundreds of diets, supplements and medications and literally thousands of books on this topic? Doesn't it stand to reason that there would be only a handful of clinically effective methods to lose weight, and that all of the others would fall out of favor?

This is exactly what happens in the world of medicine. A handful of treatments are proven to be effective for a particular condition and eventually other less effective treatments fall out of favor. Many of the medications and treatment regimens that were originally prescribed as few as ten years ago are no longer the standard of care because newer medications and improved technologies have replaced them. Diets, however, have changed very little. They tweak them from time to time, but the fads roll on.

Here's yet another way to think about this issue: How could the diet industry in the United States be a multibillion-dollar industry unless customers come back again and again over the course of their lifetimes? Diets don't work. Perhaps rather than ponying up a few hundred dollars for the next *scam de jour*, we should ask why.

Can You Ever Stop?

Okay, I rest my case: Diets are generally ineffective for most people. But why don't they work? Chapter 3 provided some answers to the weight loss question, with evolution and that toxic all-you-can-eat environment putting up among the largest hurdles. There also is another barrier, almost unique to weight loss. To understand this barrier, let's take a look at some other habits that people try to change.

Ask any former cigarette smoker and they'll tell you that at some point in their life, the urge to have a cigarette went away or diminished considerably. Without fail, most former smokers tell you that they don't think about smoking that much, if at all. They also will tell you that it's easier to resist urges than before they stopped smoking.

Plus, the entire cultural environment regarding smoking is different than that of eating and it is changing more every day. Fewer people smoke now than in past years so there is less social pressure to smoke. Smoking is far less cool than it was 25 years ago. There are no television commercials promoting cigarettes. There are no longer 35 places to sit down and smoke cigarettes in the mall. Most workplaces prohibit smoking. Nobody is offering you a super value combo cigarette meal for $1.99. In fact, in most places a pack of cigarettes costs over ten dollars a pack, providing yet another deterrent. Cigarette smoking has been linked to countless diseases, and is clearly on the decline.

The story is similar in many ways for folks who have struggled with substance abuse. Although they always need to remain vigilant for setbacks, the withdrawal symptoms and the cravings for the drugs generally diminish once they've stopped using the substance.

Perhaps the most important distinction between dieting and giving up cigarettes, alcohol and other drugs is that for virtually every other unwanted behavior, the universal goal is abstinence. The goal is not to *change* the behavior; it's to *stop* the behavior. This abstinence approach doesn't work with food and eating. You can't stop eating; you have to modify it.

Herein lies the major difficulty and distinction of dieting: Modifying behavior is generally much more difficult than stopping behavior. If you were a smoker, ask yourself if you believe you would have been successful permanently sticking to five cigarettes per day. If ever you had difficulty controlling your intake of alcohol, ask yourself if you believe you would have been able to limit yourself to one or two drinks per week. Although it is possible, it is not likely.

Scam Diets

Some diets don't work because they are outright scams. No doubt you have seen a number of pills, creams, drinks and weight loss "miracle" products touted on late night television. I've heard some of the most outrageous stories of things people have done to try to lose weight. Thankfully, consumer advocates and government agencies are finally cracking down on the ridiculous claims made by the manufacturers of these magic potions and miracle pills.

People are also getting smarter, having been burned by these scams in the past. Watch the television commercials very carefully and you will see the truth zooming by on the bottom of the screen in microscopic print: "Results not typical; your results may vary," or "This product is to be used in conjunction with a reasonable diet and exercise program." By stating that results are not typical, the manufacturer of this product is reluctantly telling you that the amazing "results" achieved by the person on your television screen represent the one person out of thousands who actually achieved success with this product. Perhaps worst of all, the manufacturer rarely provides valid data demonstrating that their regimen or product is at all superior to diet and exercise or any other product (nor are they required to by law).

What is truly unfortunate is that most folks don't fare any better on the more respectable diets. Even the balanced diets and exercise regimens designed by physicians, personal trainers, nutritionists and psychologists to establish a new, healthy "lifestyle" do not work for most people over the long term.

So why do we spend millions of dollars every year on diets and various weight loss products? Why do we try the same regimens again and again? Why do we buy crazy concoctions and give operators our credit card numbers knowing the product we are purchasing is unlikely to work? Why do we attend support groups, track our calories online, and have our food delivered? The answer is because we're desperate to lose weight, and nobody seems to have a better alternative.

Wait, There's More!

So now you've been introduced to the hurdles of evolution, our 21st century environment, and the impossibility of dieting as all standing in our way to lose weight. You wouldn't think it could get any worse, right? Well, it does. Some of the most insidious barriers to losing weight are erected by those around us, and you can find out more about them in chapter 5.

5

The Heartbreak of Social Stigma

BEING OBESE STINKS! I'M SURE this is not news to you. Obese people recognize that there is both subtle and not so subtle discrimination against them. Unfortunately, most people who are of an appropriate weight don't have a clue what obese people go through every day. If you are obese, this is common knowledge to you.

What Do They Think Of Me?

Obese people are worried about others' perceptions of them in a multitude of situations. They are concerned about being judged on what they are eating in restaurants. They are concerned about what potential employers are thinking of them during an interview. They are aware that shop clerks are reluctant to assist them in clothing stores. They see the rolling eyes and hear the sighs of the person they try to sit next to on the bus or train. Many are downright terrified about what the person across the table is thinking of them during a first date.

What are the common perceptions held by thinner folks about those who are obese? Non-obese people often think of the obese as lazy, undisciplined, unmotivated, weak, sloppy, and stupid to name a few. Numerous scientific studies completed over the years have demonstrated that there is a clear and significant bias against those who are overweight. In fact, *most* people harbor negative perceptions about people who are obese. Unfortunately, many obese people have come to share this view themselves.

Many years ago a survey appeared in a women's magazine where respondents indicated that most would rather be deaf or missing a limb than be obese. A recent survey conducted by researchers at the Rudd Center for Food Policy and Obesity at Yale University found that nearly half of the 4,000 people responding said they would give up a year of their life rather than be fat. In the same study, between 15 and 30 percent said they would rather walk away from their marriage, give up the possibility of having children, be depressed, or become alcoholic rather than be obese. These types of attitudes have been replicated in surveys time and time again. Many view obesity as both a physical handicap as well as a handicap of character.

Perhaps worst of all, as with race, the stigma surrounding obesity forms instantly. You can see it and feel it as you walk in the door. The obese person already is being judged negatively and they have yet to utter a single word. Imagine what it must be like to initiate a new social interaction and you already have one strike against you. You immediately feel like you are climbing uphill and backwards. The pressure is on to turn the tide, given that you're likely starting out on the wrong foot.

Most of my patients indicate they can feel the stigma reflected in the behavior of others. The discrimination is powerful, but often subtle. Obese people will tell you that others are reluctant to ever make eye contact or smile at them, as if they're not even there! Sadly, prior to surgery many patients state that they feel "invisible." How ironic it must be to be 100 pounds overweight yet feel completely invisible! Many of my patients have told me that their greatest sorrow is the failure of others to simply treat them as a human being.

This discrimination begins early in life. Obese children are teased and bullied perhaps more than any other group of children. The playground is an emotional slaughterhouse for such kids. Many of my patients recount stories of disparaging comments by other children as well as their teachers. Overweight teenagers will tell you that they have a number of boy or girl "friends," but not boyfriends or girlfriends. As an adult, it becomes tiresome to be constantly called "big guy." And for women it's certainly worse. Society may have a place for a six-foot tall 350-pound man to be called "big guy"; you see this on television during football games every Sunday. But you'll never hear a woman tell you she was comfortable with being called "big girl," and you certainly won't see any advertisers on television give that phrase a try.

Within the workforce, discrimination is widespread although generally unchallenged. Many of my patients have felt they didn't get a job despite their qualifications, and they walked away quietly knowing why. But sometimes the stories are remarkable. Perhaps the most astounding tale of discrimination I've heard was from a young woman who was a rising star as an employee for a prominent New York City department store. Upon receiving a promotion, she was informed by her supervisor that it would be her last and that she should not make long term plans with the company if she wished to advance any further. When she queried the supervisor as to why, her supervisor's response was that she was "not the image" that the store wanted to convey.

Make no mistake, the stigma of obesity is profound and pervasive, and for almost everyone who is obese, it takes its toll. I have yet to speak with a patient considering weight loss surgery who has said that their obesity did not affect their self-esteem or self-worth.

What Do I Think of Myself?

So with all this dreadful social punishment from others, you might assume an obese person would be motivated to lose weight. Wrong! What actually happens is the stigma gets internalized, meaning the obese person begins to actually *believe* the negative evaluations being thrown at them. Ask most obese people and they'll tell you how much their self-esteem has been shattered by their inability to lose weight. As we know from chapter 2, feeling down and demoralized can lead to emotional eating. And before you know it, you put on more pounds.

Social scientists tell us that the societal purpose of social stigma is supposed to enforce conformity. What this means is that being criticized about your weight (stigma) should lead to a loss of weight (conformity). But in the case of obesity, social stigma actually backfires by causing obese people to feel demoralized, isolated, alone, and depressed, often leading them to eat more and gain weight.

Why does stigma crush instead of motivate? Well, it's because important other elements of our society have broken down. In a healthy society or social network, social stigma may sometimes motivate change, but only when the critique is constructive and accompanied by social support. When people hear that they look ugly or disgusting, or that their obesity is their fault, this is not constructive critique. When people are shunned, avoided or ridiculed, this is not social support.

What unfortunately happens is that people begin to believe what others foolishly tell them: that their obesity is their fault. That if they just used their willpower, they wouldn't have a problem. That if they would get off their butt and put in more miles on the treadmill, they could lose all that weight. Telling people these destructive things does not empower, it demoralizes. Much of this destructive critique may occur because as a society we over-idealize thinness. But this doesn't detract from the fact that obesity is a killer disease and a killer of self-esteem and quality of life.

Hope

The last three chapters have outlined why it's so hard to lose weight. I've relayed how evolution has stacked the deck against you, how the diet industry has fed you false hope, and how people around you have destroyed your self-esteem. All of this bad news can be enough to make you throw your hands up and simply shout, *Forgetaboutit!*

Before you toss this book into the recycle bin, indulge me by reading one more story.

Not too long ago, I was working as the psychologist at a cardiac rehabilitation program, treating patients who had recently experienced a major cardiac event or were at great risk for having such an event. My role was to help people make health behavior changes, including managing stress, losing a few pounds, and adopting a more active lifestyle. We were doing some good work.

I was approached by a surgeon who was founding a surgical weight loss program. She was interested in having me work with her patients both before and after surgery. Given my experience working with overweight patients and having my own struggles with weight I was skeptical that this was yet another short term miracle. It sounded too good to be true, like all of those television ads for the latest diet craze.

At the time, I had never even heard of weight loss surgery or bariatric surgery, so the surgeon explained everything. I read everything I could get my hands on. I devoured the scientific and clinical literatures on both surgical and non-surgical weight loss approaches. I eventually decided to dedicate a few hours each week to work with the surgeon and her patients.

I am no longer a skeptic. After many years working with several thousand patients, I now believe that surgery is the best method available to help most morbidly obese patients achieve significant, lasting weight loss.

Weight loss surgery is not a guarantee to achieving eternal "thinnerness," but it can be an incredibly powerful tool unlike anything else currently available, both in the medical world and on late night infomercials. At the very least, weight loss surgery deserves serious consideration for anyone who is considered morbidly obese or who's weight is significantly affecting their health and quality of life.

6

Is Surgery Right for Me?

IN THIS CHAPTER, I WILL discuss some of the questions that I ask prospective patients during their pre-surgical consultation. Many patients beat me to the punch, as these questions represent some of the more common concerns people have prior to surgery. Most patients have given the idea of surgery a great deal of consideration and have done extensive research before they reach my office. Many have stopped and started the process a few times, wanting to give the whole matter some more thought before proceeding. It is a big decision.

Most patients finally decide to pursue weight loss surgery because everything else they've tried has failed and they believe that surgery represents their only hope for lasting weight loss. Every patient I see desperately wants to lose weight. Most indicate that their primary motivation to have surgery is to eliminate health problems or prevent them from occurring in the future. In fact, a large number of patients indicate that they were referred on the direct advice of their physician. Another common reason patients pursue surgery is because their weight has caused significant impairment in their ability to function socially or psychologically, or impacts negatively on their quality of life. Obviously, all patients want the surgery to be successful.

Surgical Candidacy

During the pre-surgical evaluation, I am frequently asked, "Who is a good candidate for weight loss surgery?" Just as often, I am asked, "Who is a poor candidate for weight loss surgery?" These are excellent questions, and both are difficult to answer. There is no definitive personality type or constellation of psychological difficulties that absolutely make someone a good or bad candidate for surgery. In my opinion, the best patients are those who are completely honest with both themselves and their psychologist, and seek to identify the stumbling blocks on the path to successful long-term weight loss, even if this means postponing their decision to have surgery.

For most patients, the real function of the pre-surgical evaluation is not to rule them in or out for surgery, but rather to assess potential obstacles that could stand in the way of success after surgery. Obviously, the major objective of weight loss surgery is to help patients lose weight. There are a number of factors that can interfere with a patient's ability to achieve that objective. I am always candid with patients. I express my understanding that the person wants to have surgery because they are confident that it will be an effective means of losing weight. Then I express concerns that I uncover during the evaluation, and we discuss them and what can be done to remedy them.

If there are significant concerns, what happens most often is that a patient and I conclude that there is good reason to postpone having surgery until they are addressed. For example, if a patient is going through a separation or divorce and they recognize that the stress from this situation is affecting their eating behavior, we might agree to wait a few months until that stress subsides. Thankfully, I have had the privilege of working with very smart and insightful patients over the years. It is quite rare that I need to convince a patient of my recommendations, as they usually share my concerns. Most are perfectly willing to wait a bit if they believe that the time can be used to ensure a more successful outcome from surgery.

What follows is a sampling of some of the more important questions that you should ask prior to having weight loss surgery.

Are My Expectations From Surgery In Line With Reality?

What do you expect from surgery? When I ask people why they are having surgery, everyone initially gives me the same answer: "To lose weight." Give it another moment of thought and you'll quickly realize that you want *more* than to simply lose weight. You want all those things that you think will come from being thinner. Asked differently, "What will your weight loss buy you?" Losing weight is, in essence, a key that can unlock the doors to your expectations.

We know that most people who have undergone weight loss surgery will lose in the neighborhood of 50 to 60 percent of their excess weight. That means you will probably lose 50 to 60 pounds for every 100 pounds that you are overweight. For example, a 5'2" tall woman weighing 225 pounds prior to surgery will likely weigh in the neighborhood of 160 pounds when all is said and done.

I often ask patients what they imagine will be different when they reach their new post-surgical weight. Many laugh and say they never thought of it this way—the goal was simply to lose all that weight.

Although I am admittedly oversimplifying things, there are basically two types of surgical weight loss patients. The first group tells me that their life is generally fine and that they want to lose weight simply to keep the music playing. These patients have fulfilling lives with loved ones, successful careers, and satisfying social lives. They believe that their weight is getting in the way of their ability to enjoy certain aspects of life, or that they are concerned that one day it will. As with most obese persons, they often have physical limitations as a result of their weight, such as difficulty walking or diminished stamina. Their decision to have surgery is primarily health related. These folks generally have very reasonable expectations from surgery because they're not asking for much; they already have most of what they want. They simply want to lose weight to be able to live longer and enjoy life more fully.

The other type of patient has much higher expectations and more riding on the outcome of surgery. Their lives are missing many elements that they believe will provide them with happiness, and they hope that these things will come when they are thinner. Many of these patients are not in satisfying relationships, have few social contacts, and may have career limitations. These folks obviously have much more on the line than those in the first group. Without question, losing weight and having improved self-esteem can make dating, job hunting and making friends a bit easier, although such results are hardly automatic.

Some folks have excessively rosy expectations, erroneously believing that life after surgery will be much easier than in actuality. For example, many patients look forward to a return to dating after they lose the weight. However, some have lost the skills of dating and are anxious about their bodies and how others would perceive them when they are thinner. In addition, potential romantic partners certainly won't just be raining out of the sky. On the other hand, some patients have more realistic expectations. When they lose the weight, they correctly understand that there is still the work of identifying new ways of meeting people such as joining groups, taking classes, and other strategies.

I will be the first to admit that I have seen patients who have been almost reborn after surgery. They lost the weight and (I'm going to get corny here) a beautiful butterfly emerges from the cocoon and goes forward to live a much happier life. These are the patients whose stories we love, the one's whose lives are truly turned around, the ones you see on television or read about in magazines. These are the patients who are rescued from their obesity and go on to live in a way that would never happen had it not been for surgery. For these patients, surgery is truly an outstanding opportunity.

However, there are many patients who find that losing the weight was the easy part. Now that they're thinner, they need to start doing things that they've been avoiding for years: dating, interviewing, socializing... Hello anxiety! Now you can understand why a psychologist may be involved both before and after surgery.

All I ask is that my patients have a clear and balanced set of expectations before having surgery. I don't discriminate against those who have big and bold expectations for life when they are thinner. It's great to dare to dream! My role is to ensure that their road map is a good one, and that they anticipate some of the winding curves and potential potholes further down the highway so that dreams don't become nightmares. Prior to my initial meeting with patients, some have already started psychotherapy, or have begun attending our support groups, or joined a gym, recognizing that this is going to be a marathon, not a sprint to the finish line.

Is This the Best Time For Me To Have Surgery?

There may not be a best time to have weight loss surgery, but some times are better than others. Surgery involves a commitment to change, both emotionally and behaviorally. It involves more than simply changing what you eat. The people most likely to be success-ful are those that consider surgery to be part of an overall change in lifestyle. You don't have to exercise every day and you don't have to count every calorie and be a slave to food. However, it helps if you view the surgery as a tool rather than a cure for obesity.

Timing is everything. Interestingly, what's going on in a person's life at the time they decide to have surgery is often the major rea-son they seek surgery. Consider my earlier example of patients who come for their pre-surgical evaluation during the middle of a separa-tion or divorce. Their plan is to lose the weight now as part of the process of starting over. Being thinner and healthier is often seen as a necessary first step on their agenda. By itself, this seems per-fectly reasonable—a fresh start. However, if it's a difficult divorce or an emotionally tumultuous time, surgery might best be postponed. Some patients freely admit that such emotional distress, whether it be anxiety, loneliness or otherwise, affects their eating, and generally not for the better. If this is the case, such patients could find them-selves struggling to acclimate to the surgery or even fighting against it. They've decided to have surgery, in part, to help control emotion-ally triggered eating at a time when their emotional eating is at an all-time high. Of course, the surgery could help reduce such behav-ior, but to ensure the long-term success of the surgery, wouldn't it be more prudent for this individual to seek out counseling or other support for their distress first? Or at the very least wouldn't it be best to wait a few months until things calmed down?

I have had this conversation with patients in the midst of a di-vorce, who have just lost a job, who are coping with the recent loss of a loved one, or who have had other types of major life crises. I feel for these people. As I said earlier, sometimes these situations are the impetus for the decision to have surgery—the final straw. A dear loved one who struggled for years with their obesity has recently died and you decide to have surgery because you don't want to follow in his footsteps. I applaud your courage in making this decision! But let's just take those steps a bit more slowly so that we can address your grieving and your obesity. Let's do this in a manner that better ensures that you achieve your goal of lasting weight loss. If there is a finite or semi-finite period of distress, waiting a bit and addressing these emotional issues prior to having surgery is reasonable to consider, and will turn out to have been a smart decision.

Who Should I Tell About My Plans To Have Surgery?

This is another great question and again one with no simple answer. Many of my patients have decided that they are only telling the people they feel they must inform—their romantic partner, their parents, their children, some close relatives, and maybe a few best friends. Others are comfortable with their decision and plan to tell everyone. For a number of reasons, I recommend the former.

Most people out in the world still don't know very much about weight loss surgery, but they're still perfectly willing to tell you what they think about it! If you tell 50 people that you plan to have surgery, you will hear 50 opinions, but 45 of them are the opinions of people who know next to nothing about the surgery, let alone the struggles of weight loss! Some folks might suggest that surgery is a cop out. Others might say that surgery doesn't really work or is dangerous based upon something they read in a magazine or heard about through the grapevine.

In my experience, those who ask more than a few people for their opinion about weight loss surgery are still unsure of the decision themselves and are seeking approval from others. If you find yourself in this category, it would be best for you to do some additional research and form your own opinion about weight loss surgery before asking others for their thoughts. When you have questions, ask people who are truly qualified to answer them. Having a conversation with your physician is often beneficial. Another approach would be to attend a weight loss surgery support group so that you can speak directly with people who have had the surgery. Patients generally tell me that members of such groups are the most helpful, informative and supportive of all.

Do I Have an Adequate Social Support Network?

Let's assume that you've had weight loss surgery, and you're ready to start anew. Now that surgery is over, it's time to consider how those around you will help you get back on your feet.

What is adequate support? It varies from person to person. Some individuals are pretty independent and don't want their surgery to be public. Others believe that they will need the support and encouragement of their friends and family to stay compliant with the changes required to be successful. The key is that you know who you are: the independent, self-reliant patient, or the one who wants encouragement and support.

Many people have a rich and wonderful circle of friends, who have supported them through thick and thin. For these folks, the support network is strong and will likely be adequate following surgery. For others, the social network is small, maybe just a few friends and loved ones. This may be sufficient, as well. One good, supportive friend is superior to several unreliable acquaintances.

What about those who have very little social support or are unsure how to find new sources of support? I recommend that every patient I see attend at least a few weight loss surgery support groups. Some say, "I'm not a group person." However, often the "non-group" people later tell me that the support group provided a valuable forum for support and encouragement. Some even came away with a few new friends. Where else can you find yourself in a room with 30 people who are all going through a process similar to your own? Who better to understand what you are experiencing? At the very least, by attending a few support groups you can truly decide if this is a valuable outlet for you.

For some, individual psychotherapy is also a good idea to provide more intensive assistance with social issues. Such therapy can sometimes help overcome longstanding barriers to developing healthy relationships. I have had a number of patients who were quite insightful and believed they could benefit by starting or resuming psychotherapy prior to having surgery. They find it helpful to have a supportive professional on board from the start. Others identify such an individual and keep their number on hand should the need arise after surgery.

Will I Miss the Food and Eating?

This is one of the most commonly asked questions and the answer is usually: Yes…and no. There are at least three things that you may miss after surgery. First, you may miss some of the foods that you used to eat. As you will discover, there are a number of foods that may be difficult to eat or that you shouldn't eat following surgery. For example, if you have a gastric bypass, you should avoid consuming foods high in sugar or fat, such as ice cream or chocolate. That's because they can trigger *dumping syndrome*, a condition that produces feelings of lightheadedness, sweating, nausea or other symptoms. If you have a laparoscopic adjustable gastric band (sometimes just called a gastric band), you may need to avoid consuming chicken breast or doughy breads that can trigger regurgitation. Comprehensive details about the required changes in eating behavior for each type of surgery are beyond the scope of this book. It's best to consult your surgeon for the requirements that apply to your own unique circumstances.

A second thing you may miss is the ability to let loose at an all-you-can-eat buffet or a wedding or holiday party. Most patients tell me that it is physically impossible to consume large quantities of food in one sitting as they could prior to surgery. Surgery will dramatically diminish the capacity of your stomach.

Third, you may miss some specific behaviors that surround the very act of eating. For a number of folks, there is strong propensity to enjoy the act of eating, and the very behaviors of chewing and swallowing can be soothing. The manner in which you will be eating (slowly with much more chewing) will feel awkward for a while until you get used to it.

In my experience, these changes alone are unlikely to trigger an episode of severe depression. In fact, I cannot recall a single patient telling me that the eating changes required by surgery resulted in feelings of severe depression where mood and level of functioning were significantly impaired. Rather, patients generally recount the positive feelings they have from being able to control the quantity they eat, while still receiving satisfaction from being able to eat the variety of foods they desire. For most folks, these positive feelings make up for missing the manner of eating, or the types and quantity of food they ate prior to surgery.

Yes, there are some folks that have difficulty making the adjustment after surgery because of the enormous role that food and eating plays in their life. In my experience, these difficulties are more common for people who eat in response to emotional distress, and this certainly needs to be considered prior to surgery. But there are tools to combat emotional eating, and these will be addressed in chapter 8.

Am I Truly Ready to Make Eating a Non-Event?

Many patients believe that they love eating and love food, and that this was a major contributor to their weight gain. Large numbers of patients tell me that they are "foodies" and that eating and cooking and thinking about food take up way too much of their time. *After surgery, this is going to change.* Being ready to make eating a non-event means that you are willing to have all things related to food take up a much smaller amount of your time.

After surgery, many people are relieved to find that eating is no longer an intimidating, anxiety-provoking process. Eating becomes more about refueling than indulging. For many, the experience of eating changes. Consider how restaurants and food critics often use the phrase "dining experience." After surgery, that "experience" will be about the ambience of the restaurant, the company you are with, and the taste and quality of the food, rather than the quantity consumed. You will need to eat slower. You will need to chew more. You will need to learn to love those precious few bites, rather than the experience of cleaning the plate.

For most of my patients, this is more of a relief than a problem. Nevertheless, it is something for which you should prepare. Summer barbecues will not be torture, but it will take some time to adjust from eating larger quantities of food to consuming only a few bites of one or two items. At a wedding where there are ten different types

of appetizers, you'll need to select only one or two because it is unlikely that you can sample all ten.

Someone who is truly ready to make eating less of an event is
acknowledging that they may miss the food on occasion, but that
they're willing to do so to obtain the positive benefit of weight loss.

Part II
Learned Eating

This section introduces the concept of learned eating. We'll learn all about the behavior of eating, such as what makes us want to eat (hunger and cravings) and why we eat in response to our emotions. Some of the controversies around viewing food as an addiction will be explored. Finally, we'll investigate the causes and consequences of binge eating, along with learning strategies that'll move you toward healthy eating behaviors.

7

Will I Still Be Hungry?

THIS IS THE TEN MILLION-DOLLAR question. Of all the concerns weight loss surgery patients have, this is perhaps the one that causes the greatest anxiety. For many, a primary reason for pursuing weight loss surgery is to gain control over eating behavior, and hunger is seen as the crucial determinant in this process. Similarly, the concept of having a surgery that controls one's eating, but not necessarily one's desire to eat, can be frightening. It would seem torturous to have a surgery that inhibits one's ability to eat, but did nothing to curtail the desire to eat.

So what's the answer to this critical question?

Thankfully, most patients that I've spoken with find that their hunger is greatly diminished following surgery. Many tell me they are rarely hungry or that the intensity of their hunger following surgery is quite manageable. However, this question is far more complex than it may seem. The difficulty in answering this question involves distinguishing hunger from craving. Some make a distinction between head hunger and stomach hunger, but they're really talking about discriminating between hunger and craving.

Hunger versus Craving

Hunger is a complex phenomenon, but it generally involves a physiological state of food deprivation. It is your brain saying: "Feed me! I need fuel!" Hunger is not particularly concerned with which specific foods are eaten in order to be satisfied. Just like your car doesn't really care if you give it Shell or Mobil gasoline, hunger doesn't really care about its fuel source.

A *craving* is a desire to eat, often for a specific food. Cravings are learned. Cravings say: "Feed me Chinese food!" or "I want M&M's." The real difficulty in recognizing and controlling cravings is that they often occur outside of your awareness. You suddenly want to eat but you're not sure why. However, there is usually a discernible reason. It's rarely a coincidence. When we can't quite understand whether cravings or hunger are foremost at play, we may become confused and attribute our wanting to eat to hunger. Adding to this confusion is that hunger and cravings influence each other. When you are hungry, your brain will focus your attention on food acquisition and you will likely think of food more often because you need food for survival. Similarly, when you see a commercial on television for corn chips, you will likely start to think about eating and may crave corn chips. And you might even begin to salivate, which is your body's way of preparing to eat. The advertising geniuses during the Super Bowl know what they're doing!

Here's an example that you've likely experienced that demonstrates the distinction between hunger and cravings. You're walking through the food court of a large shopping mall, contemplating what to have for lunch. You're clearly hungry, but your desires rapidly change from sushi to a hot dog to pizza to a burrito to a Greek salad inside of a few seconds! Behold the power of cravings. Hunger is your brain saying, "Feed me!" Cravings influence what's on your mind's menu.

You've likely heard the advice to avoid going food shopping when you're hungry. The basis for this suggestion is that hunger will encourage you to buy food to satisfy the feeling of deprivation. Cravings will encourage you to buy everything that looks or tastes good. If you go into the market hungry with the intention of only picking up a few items, you will likely come home with a cart full of goodies or impulse buys.

Learned Eating

One of the most important concepts to understand for successful weight loss is how our cravings develop. Unlike hunger, which is primarily a rudimentary biological drive, craving is more psychological and develops gradually over our life span through a process I call *learned eating*.

We *learn* to eat based upon a number of factors that we pick up rather quickly. As infants, we cry when we are hungry. Infants probably don't know what this feeling is or how to get rid of it, but they do know that it is quite unpleasant. In the uterus there is no eating, given that we receive nutrients we need directly through the umbilical cord. After birth, infants seem to have an innate ability for breast-feeding. They don't need to read any instruction manual; they just go! When are presented with a breast after birth, they turn toward it and begin to feed. If a child is being breast-fed or even formula fed, the menu is very limited but probably fully satisfying. Once real food enters the picture, things get more complicated.

Infants certainly have some rudimentary food preferences (such as strained peaches over strained asparagus!). And based on their facial expressions, newborns seem to like sugar but hate bitter flavors. Despite these preferences, the business of eating remains fairly simple. As childhood progresses, eating becomes increasingly complex. Our parents encourage us to eat certain foods and discourage us from eating others. We learn to eat because it's a specific time (lunchtime) or because we are in a certain place (the mall). We may be given food for desired behaviors, such as going potty or achieving good grades. We are comforted from emotional pain with chicken soup or chocolate chip cookies. We have a big cake on our birthday.

Our culture begins to strongly influence our food choices. What we eat depends on whether we are of Spanish, Italian, Jewish, Irish, Asian, German or African descent. Children raised in a traditional Greek home will likely develop cravings for moussaka, whereas children raised in China will likely grow up craving fish, and sticky rice.

It's important to understand that you can't possibly crave what you have never tasted. You need to *learn* the food first, and this is what learned eating is about. I never craved baklava before I first tried it, and I've never stopped craving it since! And where are we most likely to learn about our food likes and dislikes as children? If you were looking for a way to blame (or give credit to) your parents, now's the time, for the answer is your parents.

By the time we're five years old, we've probably viewed thousands of advertisements encouraging us to eat sweet, high fat goodies, 48-ounce sugary sodas, and supersized greasy burgers with French fries. Vegetables are rarely advertised. In only a short while, the business of food has turned from natural fruits, vegetables, and whole foods to chemically designed processed foods. And these processed foods are engineered to take advantage of our body's ability to engage in learned eating. The food industry creates new markets by teaching us new cravings. Unfortunately, these new foods are not always good for us.

Although both hunger and cravings will likely be diminished following weight loss surgery, cravings will not completely disappear. This is why surgery is best viewed as a tool rather than a cure to treat obesity. Case in point: A patient named Janet told me that she continued to crave peanuts following surgery, but only while she was watching television at night in her family room. She explained that she had been eating peanuts in front of the television on most nights for over 20 years! Her gastric band can't undo 20 years of learned eating. Janet will need to use other tools after surgery. And these tools involve making a number of behavior changes to maximize the long-term success of surgery.

The Science of Craving

So how do cravings get so strong? As previously mentioned, cravings are learned or conditioned. They develop through a process called classical conditioning and are maintained primarily through another process called operant conditioning. In classical conditioning, two situations, behaviors or emotions become linked with each other such that the presence of one signals that the other is coming. In a series of famous experiments, Ivan Pavlov discovered that by repeatedly pairing the ringing of a bell with the presentation of food, a dog eventually would salivate to the sound of the bell, even when there was no food. The ringing of the bell quickly became the signal or trigger letting the dog know that food was on its way. Because of this, the dog's body learned to salivate, which is a physiological response that prepares the mouth for eating.

In the case of Janet, *watching television in the den in the evening* was paired with *eating peanuts* on thousands of occasions, until eventually watching television in the den triggered a craving for peanuts. The producers of advertisements are aware of the power of classical conditioning, which is why they make commercials showing beautiful people having a great time while enjoying their products. This is also why they package toys with their children's meals. We come to associate beauty and having fun with eating a burger and fries, with little or no regard for these foods' limited nutritional value.

In operant conditioning, the performance of a specific behavior becomes strengthened due to its pleasant consequences or weakened because of its unpleasant consequences. We eat chocolate because it tastes delicious (a positive consequence) and don't eat Brussels sprouts because they don't taste very good (at least not to me!). Sometimes we eat because eating helps us escape from or cope with an unpleasant situation such as loneliness or stress (also a pleasant outcome). Like classical conditioning, operant conditioning occurs hundreds of time every day, mostly outside of our awareness, and it has extremely powerful influences on our behavior.

Our consumption of *comfort foods* provides an example of both types of conditioning at work. We are classically conditioned to associate certain foods with certain people (grandma with cookies) or happy times (childhood with sweets). These foods tend to be delicious foods (a positive consequence). After eating comfort foods thousands of times, we learn to crave these foods during times when we need an emotional pick-me-up or comfort. Our brain links specific foods with specific desired emotional outcomes. It's as if your brain reminds you: "Hey you, the guy feeling lonely and blue, go get some cookies—they'll make you feel better!"

Control Your Cravings

Learning to control your cravings is crucial to enhance your success after weight loss surgery. The best way to *unlearn* old cravings is to *recondition* yourself by learning new ways of thinking and behaving to replace the habit of eating when the old craving trigger is pulled.

Conditioning in real life usually involves multiple triggers that can set off a craving for food. And triggers take many forms, such as a feeling, a place, or a time of day. Social triggers may also be in the mix, where some people may be a greater trigger than others. Even the absence of people (being alone) can be a trigger. When enough of these triggers are pulled, this could set up a strong enough craving that prompts you to eat.

For example, you might notice that when you're in a bad mood, alone, in your den, at night, you eat nacho chips. Here you've got four very powerful triggers (a feeling, the absence of people, a place, and a time) that in the past may have been associated with eating nachos. Now put them all together at once and you start eating.

The first step to defeat your cravings involves identifying the triggers that set them off. Eventually you'll need to replace those triggers with new, non-triggering events. And you'll need to replace the unhealthy eating behavior with new healthy behaviors. Here are some suggestions to get you started:

- ✓ Begin by keeping a *diary* of your cravings. If you're going to be successful in changing your behavior, you first need to become aware of patterns in your current behavior. You can use the blank *Cravings Diary Worksheet* in appendix B.

- ✓ Document your *triggers*, such as when and where you had the craving and what food you craved. See if you can identify specific triggers for your cravings. Where you eat, when you eat, and whom you're with can all be potential triggers. The craving diary may also teach you that specific people, places, emotions, or situations trigger your cravings.

- ✓ Distinguish *hunger versus craving*. Sometimes just recognizing that you are experiencing a craving rather than hunger is effective in giving you control to resist the urge to eat. Knowing that you are not really hungry makes it easier to tell your body that will have to wait. Remind yourself that you want to eat, but don't need to eat.

✓ Practice your ability to *resist the cravings* by either not eating, eating smaller portions, or eating healthier alternative
foods. If you actively practice such resistance, you'll be
able to prove to yourself that resistance is not futile!

As you begin to fill in your craving diary over the course of a
few weeks, some patterns will begin to emerge. You'll begin to see
those triggers that are most often associated with your eating. It may
be the mood, the location or a combination of factors that seems to
provoke the desire for peanuts or nacho chips.

Now I know what you're thinking: I hate writing down what I
eat. The primary reason that most people hate writing down what
they eat is that it forces them to be accountable for their behavior.
And with this comes the discomfort of acknowledging what you're
eating. Then you're left with a choice: Change what you're eating or
recognize that you're eating what you know you shouldn't be eating.
By documenting your behavior, you learn what triggers prompt your
eating. Only by knowing these triggers will you be able to make the
necessary changes in your behavior. Without writing it down, you're
just winging it, and I guarantee you that those wings will take you
nowhere.

Perhaps the most difficult part of changing your behavior is developing the ability to recognize unwanted behaviors at the moment
they are about to occur. It's as if you need to press the pause button
on the world around you to stop what you're doing and behave in a
different manner. The reason for this is that much of our behavior
occurs outside of our awareness, while running on autopilot. This
is why I am telling you to drop those wings and switch out of autopilot!

Habit Strength and Mindless Eating

There comes a point where it appears that the chips and peanuts
are calling you to come and get them rather than you making a decision to go and get them. Every time you eat peanuts and nacho chips
in front of your television while feeling bored and lonely increases
the likelihood that you will do it again in the future, given the same

circumstances, and especially if it feels good. This tendency for a be-havior to become stronger and more automated through repetition is called *habit strength*.

Think of habit strength as our brain being set to autopilot on a plane or the default setting of a computer. We gradually become programmed to engage in the behavior of eating under a certain set of circumstances and often do it subconsciously. This is called *mindless eating*.

There's a good chance that your surgery will take the edge off of your hunger. Many people who have had surgery report that they still crave the foods they've always enjoyed, but that the strength of the cravings is lower. Prior to surgery, these same patients have told me that their cravings feel like an impossibly strong desire that can-not be ignored. Hopefully, you will find your cravings diminish as a result of surgery. But they will not disappear! You will still need to combat mindless eating by bringing those cravings into awareness and doing something about them, even if that something is learning to tolerate the discomfort of wanting to eat while you choose to look the other way.

Attacking Your Cravings

So now you know that you need to switch out of autopilot and stop that mindless eating to become better aware of the situations or circumstances surrounding your cravings. But once you are aware of your cravings, how do you handle them? You've got two tools at your disposal:

1. *Avoid* the situation.
2. *Alter* your behavior.

A combination of both is optimal because you cannot live a life that exclusively calls upon only one of these strategies. You cannot avoid each and every situation that causes cravings. And you may find it difficult to alter your behavior in some circumstances. Most situations call for a combination of avoiding and altering.

Earlier in this chapter you've discovered some of the triggers for your cravings with the *Cravings Diary Worksheet*. Your next step is to make changes in how you respond to those cravings. These changes will involve either making new food choices or discovering new behaviors to replace eating entirely. In appendix B you'll find the *Eating Alternatives Worksheet* to get started.

This worksheet will help you generate new adaptive behaviors that serve as a healthy alternative to eating. Then you can try those new behaviors when you experience cravings. When you have an urge to eat, keep track of what you tried to do instead of eating, and whether this method helped you overcome your craving. Sometimes it will; sometimes it won't. By trying different alternatives to eating, you will learn that you don't have to succumb to your cravings. More importantly, you will develop new and healthy habits that break the impulse to eat in response to every craving.

If you find that loneliness triggers cravings, explore opportunities for increased social activity: Call a friend, go online, sign up for a class, go to the mall, or do something else that puts you in a new social environment. Anything that involves other people is better than sitting alone in your living room.

If nighttime television watching appears to be the trigger, participate in other activities during the evenings, particularly ones that are incompatible with eating. Exercising is a perfect example. Not only is exercise something new to do, it's something that you *can't* do while you eat. As a result, it further promotes the goals of weight loss and wellness. Consider joining a gym or creating a regimen of exercise that you can stick with. One of my patients put an elliptical trainer square in the middle of her living room in front of the television as a reminder that she is supposed to use it at least a few nights per week.

If you find that boredom triggers your cravings, you must first weaken the link between boredom and the behavior of eating. Then you must create new links in the chain by doing new, fun, and interesting things that compete with boredom, and ultimately eating. Explore new interests to keep you busy. There's a big wide world out there, and many new activities to consider.

There is a special class of triggers for which eating can sometimes have an especially strong positive consequence, and these triggers are called negative emotions. When eating soothes our bad feelings, and when this occurs repeatedly so that we begin to rely on significant amounts of food to help us feel better, this is called *emotional eating*. Essentially, food is being used as a medication. This association between emotional triggers, craving, and the resultant learned eating is an especially strong one, and we explore it more fully in our next chapter.

8

How Do I Tackle Emotional Eating?

THIS IS ONE OF THE more commonly asked questions prior to surgery. Pure and simple, *emotional eating* is the consumption of food in response to how you feel, and it's one form of *learned eating*. There is considerable anxiety about how emotional eating might affect the success of surgery. In this chapter, we'll explore emotional eating in great detail to help you think more rationally about addressing such anxiety. In fact, it's a good idea to begin managing emotional eating *before* having surgery.

To some degree, it's important to normalize emotional eating. Everyone eats in response to emotions and therefore we are all emotional eaters to some extent. Eating is an inherently emotional phenomenon. That's because hunger, appetite, and cravings are all controlled by areas of the brain that are also involved in our experience of emotions. Moreover, there are long-standing patterns of behavior where we're all trained to eat in response to certain feelings or occasions.

Two Types of Emotion

The entire spectrum of emotions can be divided into two very broad categories: positive emotions and negative emotions. Positive emotions include happiness, joy, pride, and so on. Negative emotions include depression, loneliness, anger and anxiety.

Positive emotions—let's celebrate!

Almost everyone has experienced eating in response to positive emotions. Could you imagine a child's birthday party without a birthday cake? Similarly, for most of us it's hard to imagine Thanksgiving without the turkey. Aren't these examples of emotional eating? Many people celebrate certain occasions by going out for dinner. What child isn't filled with joy at the prospect of going out for hamburgers and French fries and then to the ice cream shop? Similarly, many people have sent and received baskets of fruit or food as gifts. Emotional eating is a common part of most cultural and religious traditions, some more than others. Can you imagine Thanksgiving, Christmas, Passover, Easter or Hanukkah without the special foods we associate with them? It wouldn't be the same at all, would it?

In excess, this form of emotional eating can be a problem and we could all stand to learn a bit of restraint on holidays and in our celebrations. But completely terminating the eating part of the celebration isn't a reasonable suggestion, either. Most patients have confided that after surgery they continued to enjoy eating as part of such festivities, but that the amount of food consumed was smaller. The summertime backyard barbecue, for example, is now one hot dog and some salad rather than two hot dogs, a hamburger and lots of potato salad.

Negative emotions—food, the ultimate antidepressant.

Think of negative emotions as the painful feelings we wish to avoid. They include depression, anxiety, worry, sorrow, loneliness, among others. Sometimes they are mild and other times they are severe. Concern can be considered a mild form of worry. Disappointment is a mild form of depression. The popular definition of emotional eating posits that there is an underlying source of emotional distress that the individual is attempting to "medicate" with food, hence the term *self-medication*.

The relationship between appetite and emotions is very complex. Sometimes people experience an increase in appetite when they are distraught and other times they lose their appetite. Sometimes people eat in response to minor negative emotions and other times they eat in response to major negative ones. Knowing which type you experience and becoming more aware of your emotion–eating connection will help you minimize the effect your emotions have on eating, and ultimately your weight.

For example, many folks remember *losing weight* after the breakup of a long-term relationship or following the death of a dear loved one, recalling that they simply had no appetite. In contrast, others can recall "blowing" their diet and *gaining weight* following a similar event. When I review diet histories with patients prior to surgery, they commonly cite a negative emotional event (death of a parent, loss of job, breakup of a relationship) as the incident that caused a particular diet to unravel and for weight gain to recur. These seemingly contradictory effects of negative emotional states on eating behavior are well documented. In fact, significant weight loss or weight gain are both common symptoms of serious depression.

Adding to the complexity of the emotion–eating relationship is that some patients report that they eat in response to mild negative emotions while others eat in response to severe negative emotions. In other words, sometimes we eat because of minor daily hassles or stressors, while other times we eat in response to major life problems or severe stress. Again, knowing your unique habits is crucial in learning how to change your own behavior.

Thankfully, life's truly terrible events do not occur that often. *For most of us, it's the daily grind of minor negative emotions that we need to watch out for.* Not surprisingly, this is what most people report as their major concern following weight loss surgery.

The Vicious Cycle

Many folks can attest to the fact that eating temporarily makes them feel better. A little less depressed…a little less anxious. Unfortunately, the relief is short lived and often compounds the problem. You may be all too familiar with the following experience:

> Imagine yourself eating a sleeve of cookies alone in your living room at night while watching television. The primary triggers for your eating are feeling lonely, sad and a bit hopeless. After consuming a few cookies, you begin to feel angry with yourself for binging like this, yet again.
>
> Now you're angry and decide to finish the sleeve because at this point you feel like it doesn't matter anymore. You've already had 1,000 calories worth of cookies, so what difference does it make that you consume another 250? With that discovery, you now feel even more lonely, sad and hopeless.

This example illustrates the vicious cycle that links cravings with emotional eating. The diagram on the next page outlines the steps of this cycle. The trigger that starts the cycle is emotional upset (step 1). The person begins to eat (step 2) and feels some temporary relief from the distress. However this relief is short-lived, replaced by feelings of guilt about a return to eating (step 3). This bad feeling of guilt blends together with earlier feelings of sadness, causing the person to eat even more (step 4) in an attempt to seek relief from these negative emotions. This eating once again provides some temporary relief, though it is quickly replaced by more intense negative emotions, with feelings of hopelessness about ever being able to stop eating and consequent self-loathing (step 5). Next, you guessed it, more eating ensues to soothe the bad feelings, and the vicious cycle continues.

Ironically, the person in our example has "learned" that they can experience a brief sense of relief from feelings of loneliness by engaging in a lonely and self-defeating behavior! How can that possibly be helpful? It is not. But the person in our example has an autopilot that is set to eating under these circumstances. Therefore, she would be best served by doing just about *anything other than eating*, just to begin to break the cycle. You don't have to know for certain what behavior would be better. All you have to know is that doing the same thing over and over again *can't* be helpful. So anything else is a step in the right direction.

Imagine if this same person decided to join a binge eating group that meets in the evening. That could be helpful. It's outside the

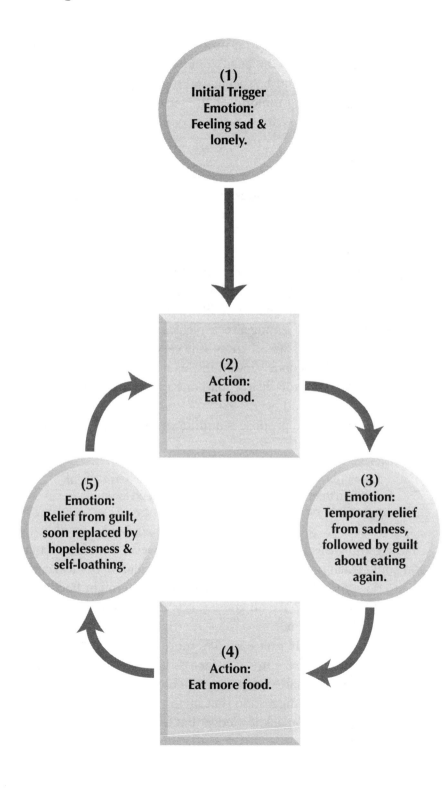

home, it's a social activity, and it probably would not involve much eating. Similarly, going to the gym would be appropriate. Again, it's away from home, it could be social, and it certainly doesn't involve eating. The key is being mindful of the vicious cycle and finding a new behavior to replace eating. Keep an open mind and possibilities become clearer.

With Friends Like These, Who Needs Enemies?

At first, breaking this vicious cycle of emotional eating can feel quite overwhelming. Some have told me it's like losing a relationship with a close, dear friend. What will I do without my "good old friend" food?

But don't you think it's rather *strange* that an overweight person would consider food to be a friend? Most friends don't damage your health or diminish your quality of life. The problem again is that the *immediate* effects of eating are a pleasant taste and a pleasant emotional state. And as we all know, it is very difficult to stop doing what *immediately* feels good. Viewed in this way, food is not a "good old friend" at all. It's more like a "bad one night stand," except that you are doing it over and over.

What I am going to propose is admittedly an oversimplification, but please listen carefully:

> Defeating emotional eating boils down to increasing your frustration tolerance and minimizing your need for *immediate* gratification.

Now I know this isn't a popular idea. However, isn't it true that if you could learn to tolerate your emotional upset and not feel compelled to do something right now to feel better you might be able to put those Oreos down? We all know this is the truth, but have such a hard time just saying no.

And I'll admit it: It isn't easy. It's more complicated than just saying no, and there are numerous factors involved that go beyond willpower. What has made you angry when people have said this to you in the past is their suggestion that saying no is the *entire* solution. All I'm asking is that you acknowledge that learning to tolerate some discomfort is *part* of the solution. Later in this chapter I'll provide some more concrete steps for managing your emotional eating.

Mindless Eating

Making matters worse is the fact that most emotional eating is often done in a mindless fashion, or what some folks call *mindless eating* or *unconscious eating*. I briefly discussed mindless eating in chapter 7. It's very hard to change a behavior that you're not even aware you're doing! Most people generally don't actively think: Gee, I'm really nervous about my exam tomorrow; maybe some pretzels would help with my anxiety. Instead, they plop down on the couch with their books and a bag of pretzels and voila! In ten minutes the bag is empty.

Here's the problem: Long-standing repeated patterns of behavior like eating become automatic and ultimately occur without our awareness. Many of the things we do like breathing, walking, driving, typing, and eating can be performed without much awareness—and sometimes completely without awareness. Have you ever driven to a common destination and suddenly realized that you couldn't remember any of the details of the trip? You've driven this route thousands of times, so your brain stored the details of the trip on autopilot. This makes it easier for you to attend to other matters, like thinking about work while driving. In many cases, the brain's propensity for storing common behaviors on autopilot can be quite helpful, except when it comes to eating; then, this tendency can be quite dangerous.

How many times can you remember sitting in front of the television eating cookies or chips straight out of the bag? And then you went to fish your hand into the bag for another handful, only to find that the bag was empty. Often you can't even remember eating more than one or two handfuls! Could I possibly have eaten an entire bag of potato chips without being aware of it? Yes! How many times have you mindlessly consumed four pieces of bread that were sitting in the basket on the table in your favorite Italian restaurant before you even got your salad? It's the same phenomenon.

Two culprits are usually behind mindless eating: *boredom* and *habit*. We've all done this and it illustrates how easily and willingly our brains put eating on autopilot. Many admit that they are not the least bit hungry when they eat in this manner. Eating is simply something to do—and we do it over and over, making it a habit. One of the most common emotions that triggers mindless eating is boredom. We've got nothing better to do, so we eat.

The antidote for this form of emotional eating is to become more mindful by giving eating more than a passing thought. Doing so simply means that you are paying attention and that your thoughts focus on what you are doing. You *redirect attention* to what you are doing, and this makes you aware of eating. One helpful strategy is to confine eating to specific times and places so that you can't just kick into autopilot. If you eat only a few times a day and only in a few places, it is far easier to keep track of your behavior and you'll be less likely to slip. Another strategy is to bring a predetermined amount of food to the television room, such as only a handful of pretzels instead of the entire box, to prevent autopilot from encouraging you to finish off the bag.

One way to avoid mindless eating is to consciously limit your behavior to only one activity. If you're driving, don't eat, and certainly don't drink. If you're watching a movie, don't munch on popcorn. Because mindless eating often occurs while you are doing something else, making a conscious effort to stick to one activity can often help. You've probably heard these suggestions before, but perhaps now you understand them better in this context.

It's critical that you avoid mindless eating if you are going to lose the most weight from weight loss surgery. The worst mistake you can make is to assume that your surgery will stop this behavior for you. If you do, old habits will creep right back in and send your weight moving in the wrong direction. Surgery cannot stop mindless eating—only *you* can.

The Dangerous Stew

The real danger is when mindlessness and severe emotional eating converge. This type of eating happens most often at home in the evening, possibly because most people feel uncomfortable overeating at work and also because the evening is often the least structured part of the day. Evening is when we unwind and let our hair down and act like who we really are, not who we show the world at work. Evening can also be when our emotions come out to play.

A number of single people share with me that they have an evening eating ritual triggered by loneliness. Others indicate that they eat in the evening to cope with their worries, while still others report that eating is simply a way to unwind at the end of a difficult day. Many who eat at night view this behavior as a well-deserved "reward" for tolerating the rigors of a hard day. Using food as a reward is a dangerous mix. Here we have the convergence of all our evils into one dangerous stew: boredom, emotional distress, habit, and mindlessness.

Interestingly, under these conditions ice cream is a remarkably common choice. I've observed that ice cream is primarily consumed at night, except perhaps for weekends and summertime. Have you ever seen an adult eating ice cream during the workday? It's not common.

Going it Alone

If your emotional eating is minor and you don't see a major impact on your weight or on your mind, you might want to try addressing the problem yourself. If so, there are numerous books on emotional eating you can consult. In fact, you already have. Most approaches incorporate some form of *self-monitoring*. How can you begin to change your behavior before you completely understand what it is that you are changing? After gaining an understanding of some of the triggers for your emotional eating, it becomes a matter of making small and incremental changes in your behavior, both in terms of better managing the emotions that trigger eating as well as finding alternatives to the eating behavior.

To begin self-monitoring, the first thing you need to do is to pull out that *Cravings Diary Worksheet* we discussed in chapter 7. A copy is available for you to use in appendix B. Keep this diary for about three to five weeks, and complete it by focusing primarily on the *mood triggers* for your eating. In your diary, document every instance of emotional eating, the situation that triggered it, what you were thinking and feeling when it occurred, and what you ate. Forget about calorie counting; that's not important here. What you are trying to do is uncover patterns in your emotional eating. After a few weeks of this form of self-monitoring you will have some valuable information about the emotional triggers for your eating behavior.

Complete your diary in a nonjudgmental, observational manner. At this point, your goal is to learn about the immediate factors that contribute or cause you to eat *beyond* hunger. What seems to be triggering you to go to the fridge or the pantry? You cannot begin to fix a problem until you evaluate and understand its complexities. An auto mechanic doesn't start tinkering with an engine until he looks and listens underneath the hood. And that's exactly what I'm asking you to do.

As you complete your diary this time, you'll be focusing specifically on your emotional triggers for eating. These are the things you would write in the "What am I feeling? What mood am I in?" column. Over time, you'll notice that there are probably a small set of emotions that make a regular appearance. For example, you might keep seeing "lonely" or "stressed." If so, you'd need to determine how you are going to address your loneliness or high levels of stress by doing something other than eating. If loneliness is your mood trigger, you'll need to start taking steps to form some new relationships. If stress keeps reappearing, you'll need to begin exploring and implementing some stress management strategies. In this way you can begin to develop a repertoire of new behaviors to address those emotions that trigger your eating.

Focus On the Present

I *strongly* encourage you to keep your focus on the *here and now*. Avoid saying negative things to yourself about this eating problem. Don't be lulled into trying to "figure it all out." This is a trap! We are all fascinated with trying to understand the deep, hidden roots of our behavior to learn where things originated. But even when we *think* we know, we don't *really* know. Worst of all is that trying desperately to analyze the past serves as a distraction from making difficult but achievable behavioral changes in the present. While understanding some of the bigger "why" questions may have some benefits, it's not relevant here. Remember this:

> Knowing where and why your eating problem began in the *distant past* is not necessary for you to make significant behavior changes in the *present*.

The belief that uncovering your distant past solves the problem is unfortunately a widely believed myth. Interestingly, even when you do have an understanding of the circumstances that gave rise to your eating problem, having this information itself does not make the problem disappear. In fact, it can distract you. This is called *magical thinking*. Here's an example:

> During a recent psychotherapy session with a patient struggling with binge eating, I was able to help her recognize that her frequent craving for Chinese food was not random. She was able to understand that loneliness triggered an urge to eat, particularly on weekends. What she couldn't immediately understand is *why* her cravings were always for Chinese food and *why* on weekends?
>
> Through our discussion, she realized that her family commonly ate dinner in a Chinese restaurant on Sunday night when she was a child, and that this meal was one of the few times her parents were able to get along without fighting. She also recognized that these Sunday night dinners might have been the only time when her family actually felt like a family. It was a time when family spoke to one another in a calm, pleasant manner. The food was hardly the important part of the gathering. For her, eating Chinese food was associated with calmness, pleasantries, and love. So for her, the history of eating Chinese food was a way to cope with loneliness by connecting to these positive memories from childhood.
>
> Voila! She thought she was done! This explanation made my patient feel less freakish about her binging on Chinese food on most weekends. However, *it did little to change her behavior in the present.* Her binge eating continued to be an issue that we needed to address in the therapy.

Again, the reason I encourage you to avoid getting stuck on answering the big "why" questions is that they distract and delay you from making achievable gains in the present. Much progress can be made in changing your behavior, even if we never learn where the problem came from. Consider that in the world of medicine, most treatments are quite successful even though we may never learn the origin of the disease. You don't need to know which child in your child's class gave him the flu. You only need to correctly diagnose his illness and give him the appropriate medications to treat it.

Getting Extra Help

This whole emotional eating business can be quite complex. If you find that you are struggling after trying to go it alone, I strongly encourage you to find a mental health professional such as psychologist or social worker who specializes in binge eating or eating disorders, and preferably someone who is well informed about weight loss surgery. A good professional can be tremendously helpful in providing information and support as you try to tackle emotional eating.

The patient I described above is a good example of someone who may need extra help. Most of the patients I treat are very bright, motivated and insightful, fully capable of reading self-help books or buying patient-guided treatment manuals. However, all have commented about how difficult it was to hold themselves to task, trying to stay on target week after week. And many have said that it's even harder to be objective with themselves about their feelings and behaviors. So don't fret. If you feel you need the extra help, get it!

Beyond Emotional Eating

There are two common concerns among those who eat in response to their emotions. First, there is a fear that they might turn to another self-destructive behavior to replace eating, such as drinking alcohol, using drugs, gambling, or excessive spending. Second, many folks may have experienced the reverse: They recall having gained a significant amount of weight after they stopped smoking, possibly substituting food for the cigarettes, either to help cope with stress of quitting or simply as a behavior that replaced smoking. Still others have not experienced these problems first hand, but have heard such stories through the media.

Although these concerns of one problem behavior leading to another are not unfounded, they don't always represent a certainty. We'll explore this idea in the next chapter.

9

Am I Addicted to Food?

I CAN'T TELL YOU HOW many times I've heard this question, in one form or another. Patients, professionals, people on the street, all wondering whether it is possible to be addicted to food. The desire to embrace an addiction model when it comes to eating has numerous influences. The prevalence of self-help groups like Overeaters Anonymous, the strength of the addiction disease model and twelve step programs in treatment centers across the United States, and the popular moralistic tendency to view every pleasurable behavior as an addiction all contribute to the adoption of an addiction model for eating behavior.

Addiction Transfer

With regard to eating behavior, the possibility of being addicted to food has its roots in the concept of *addiction transfer* (sometimes called *cross addiction* or *symptom substitution*). Addiction transfer involves the belief that if an eating problem is successfully tackled, it inevitably will be replaced with another self-destructive behavior, like alcohol use or gambling. The question also derives from past experiences of weight gain after quitting smoking or drinking or some other unhealthy behavior. For example, some people vividly recall replacing cigarettes with M&M's, jellybeans or other types of food.

Interestingly, some of my patients who had previously battled alcohol dependence reported that members of Alcoholics Anonymous actually encouraged them to "replace" their ingestion of alcohol with sugar. Because they were engaging in a *conscious* decision to replace one behavior (drinking alcohol) with another (eating), the reasoning went, the substitution did not constitute a true "transfer" of addiction.

These experiences lead many to strongly believe that they must be addicted to food, and that they need to view food as a "drug" and see eating as a "bad behavior." The addiction view is closely related to *emotional eating* and *self-medicating* behavior, both discussed in chapter 8. Here's the logic that seems to reinforce the idea that it's possible to be addicted to food:

> If my current method of coping with emotional distress, eating, was to be prevented or sharply curtailed by weight loss surgery, I would either figure out a way to "eat around the surgery" or engage in "symptom substitution" or "addiction transfer" where I would be motivated to continue "self-medicating" with a new behavior like smoking, alcohol use, drug use, or compulsive shopping.

Boy, we sure do love our catch phrases don't we! This all sounds quite scary, and for some people there is reason for concern. But there are reasons to be hopeful, as well. In my experience, the vast majority of people who were not problematic emotional eaters before weight loss surgery do not begin engaging in this or related behaviors after surgery. I do not commonly see people suddenly indulging in foods after surgery that they didn't indulge in prior to surgery.

Those who were significant emotional eaters before surgery do need to keep an eye on their behavior to avoid difficulties following surgery, but *not* because they are addicted to food and *not* because their past excessive eating will suddenly "transfer" over to excessive alcohol use. Even among those who continue to engage in emotional eating following surgery, it is uncommon that I work with someone where this behavior has prevented significant weight loss or caused considerable weight regain.

So what's all the fuss about?

Some scientists who have conducted research on addiction transfer have found that patients with histories of binge eating or substance abuse who have weight loss surgery are at risk for problems with other destructive behavior such as alcohol abuse after surgery. However, other researchers have not found this phenomenon. The jury is definitely still out. We do not yet fully understand why some patients are at risk to adopt other maladaptive behavior patterns while others are not. And we have little understanding of the mechanism by which an individual's inability to engage in emotional eating results in their adoption of another behavior such as alcohol abuse.

The notion that one behavioral problem such as binge eating "transfers" into another such as alcohol abuse is a leap beyond the current research and is misleading. The very term "addiction transfer" is questionable and controversial.

We're All Addicts

Is eating *really* an addiction? Can we *really* be addicted to food? Are some foods "substances" similar to the way alcohol, nicotine, cocaine and heroin are substances? Is compulsive eating or binge eating a true addiction or is it more like a "soft addiction" similar to compulsive gambling or compulsive spending and shopping? These questions are the subject of great debate and boil down to how *addiction* is defined.

If addiction is primarily a physiological phenomenon, then the jury is still out. While there are studies illustrating changes in brain chemistry while engaging in some of these "soft addictions," equating compulsive shopping with cocaine abuse is a stretch. If you stretch too far, just about *anything* could be deemed an addiction, like watching too many cable television news programs. However, with drugs the substance is rather obvious as are its immediate physiological effects. Nobody questions whether or not cigarettes or heroin are addictive. But what is the "substance" when it comes to eating?

Many writers and some professionals have been trying to indict simple carbohydrates or refined sugars as the demonic substance for years; but research doesn't show this to be the case. Sugar is not the great Satan of the food kingdom. Simple carbohydrates definitely have immediate effects on blood sugar and their absence from your diet can result in cravings. But this is not quite the same process that occurs when an opiate addict is withdrawing from heroin. The carbohydrate "addiction" is still more fantasy than reality. In fact, most research suggests that people are more apt to choose high-fat foods than high-carbohydrate foods so fatty foods are perhaps more addictive than sugary ones, if you insist on applying the concept of addiction.

Our propensity to eat when stressed almost assuredly has a biological basis. But that biology intimately interacts with the environment to produce psychological (emotions, thoughts) and behavioral outcomes. A good body of scientific research has demonstrated the following sequence of events when any of us experience stress:

1. An alarming or fearful situation is perceived as a threat.

2. The "fight or flight" response is activated, where the organism has a strong immediate motivation to either remain in the situation and address the threat or leave the situation.

3. Stimulation of the hypothalamic–pituitary axis.

4. Increased release of cortisol and other chemicals.

5. These chemicals, in turn, stimulate the eating of high calorie, fatty and salty foods.

6. Immediate reduction of stress.

7. Increase in likelihood that eating behavior will be repeated in the future, especially in response to stress.

This chain of events is a fairly well documented process and occurs in a matter of seconds. From this sequence, you might conclude that we are wired to eat when stressed, and you would be mostly correct. In fact, food in general is probably the original "substance," and every other substance we get hooked on is just riding those same food pleasure pathways in the brain. So if eating has this capacity to reduce stress in all of us, doesn't that make us all food addicts? Hardly!

Consider the fact that everyone *sometimes* does *something* (including eat!) to cope with negative emotions or events. Nobody sits in a chair and simply stares at the wall when they are upset. Well, very few do! Because most humans are poor at tolerating emotional discomfort, and because life at times can be quite stressful, it is no surprise that many will engage in a wide variety of behaviors to seek comfort, like gambling, eating, sex, or online shopping. Does this make them all addicts?

Why Food Addiction Is a Bad Idea

Why am I fighting so hard against calling food and eating an addiction? Funny you should ask! Well, I've got several reasons. I've already mentioned two: that the evidence on addiction transfer is equivocal, and that the drive to engage in behaviors to cope with negative events is essentially universal. There are more, related to the philosophical roadblocks that an "addiction" concept puts in the way of your weight loss success. I should mention that these road-blocks are shared by many, but not all, views of addiction. Nonetheless they are sufficiently prevalent and serve to reinforce the concept of food addiction. Let's look at each, in kind:

An addict is powerless.

One requirement that sometimes accompanies a definition of addiction is the acceptance of powerlessness. Although there are advantages to understanding that you may be powerless over some of the *causes* of your weight problem, there is a great danger that this powerlessness could generalize to your thoughts about the *solutions* of your weight problem. In my experience, the two consequences that generally follow from the belief that you are powerless over food and your eating are: (1) to *feel* hopeless, and (2) to *behave* helplessly.

When you believe that your eating behavior is hopeless because of your "addiction" to food, you start to believe that you can't do anything, and soon behave accordingly. The belief that you are powerless and the feelings of hopelessness that ensue often create a *self-fulfilling prophecy*. And holding this prophecy causes you to avoid making a consistent effort to alter your behavior. You eat a few too many cookies and feel badly about it. You start thinking:

> Why should I bother to try? I'm a "food addict," and I
> can't control myself. Screw it! I might as well just keep eat-
> ing. It's never going to change. Why even bother?

I hear patients recounting this story almost every day and it is complete nonsense. By believing that you are powerless to control yourself, you are more likely to give up and simply allow yourself to keep eating, believing that there is no solution to the problem.

There is little benefit to believing that you are powerless to change your behavior and there is absolutely no benefit in doing so. You can always make an effort to control your behavior, no matter how difficult it may be. Also consider that if you are powerless to change your behavior, then who can? Your surgeon? Your psychologist? No! It's got to be you!

An addict must abstain.

In our society, thinking of yourself as a "food addict" inevitably leads to the suggestion that you probably have a "disease" of "food addiction" from which some form of abstinence is the only rational cure. While there are some benefits to viewing morbid obesity as a disease (see chapter 2), prescribing abstinence as a solution has significant limitations.

First of all, what are we abstaining from? We again have the problem of identifying the supposed "substance" that is to be avoided. Usually it's sugar, but why not fat? Why is it in the abstinence model that chocolate bars are off limits but bacon and salami are okay? This makes no sense and over the long run would prevent lasting weight loss.

A larger problem is that most research conducted on emotional eating, compulsive eating or binge eating actually demonstrates that abstinence, in the form of radical dieting (see chapter 4), is more likely the *cause* of the problem rather than the solution. That's right: Abstaining usually leads to excessive restraint and obsessing over *forbidden* or *comfort foods*. Eventually, when you finally gain access or grant yourself permission to eat such foods, you overdo it.

If you choose to abstain from certain foods, you must believe that there are "good" foods and "bad" foods and "safe" foods and "dangerous" foods. You must believe that consuming "bad" foods is "cheating" and that maintaining your abstinence is being "good." These thoughts are all part of the mindset that gives rise to compulsive or disordered eating problems. Holding beliefs that cookies are "bad" and that someone who eats cookies is a "failure" is unfounded. And such irrational, *all-or-none* or *black-and-white thinking* is the problem, not the solution!

A better option would be to reframe the entire concept of "forbidden" foods. I suggest we refer to them as *risky foods* or *trigger foods*. This way you've got something to watch out for (a risk) instead of something to fear or avoid. You'll also provide a logical definition for what such foods can potentially do (trigger your eating). With this new thinking framework, you'll be better able to combat unhealthy eating.

An addict never learns.
Related to the notion of powerlessness and the experience of diet failure is the argument in some addiction circles that it is impossible to teach a patient new methods to lose weight. This view assumes people who are obese ultimately have no true control over their excessive eating. Some suggest that because a person repeats the same destructive behaviors over and over, she is hopelessly condemned to a life of obesity, destined to endlessly repeat the same addictive behavior.

This is rubbish! If we adopt a *learned eating* view instead of a *food addiction* view, it is entirely possible to break the emotional eating cycle and learn new behaviors.

If Eating Is Not an Addiction, What Is It?

A behavior that becomes difficult to control and comes to have negative consequences in one's life is referred to as a *compulsion*. Compulsive shoppers shop to excess, often with money they don't have and at great consequence to their financial well-being. Compulsive gamblers similarly put their financial futures in jeopardy. A compulsive eater eats quantities of food that are excessive and unhealthy.

Consuming one candy bar would not be evidence of a compulsion. Neither would be occasionally eating too much ice cream. To be truly compulsive, we need to see a repetitive, long-term pattern of destructive behavior.

To be sure, eating is highly reinforcing. This means that the wonderful tastes and emotions we experience (or gain relief from) when eating make it more likely that we'll repeat this behavior in the future, sometimes despite the ensuing negative consequences. Eating is a naturally rewarding activity, and for some folks can become difficult to curtail. What's important to recognize is that this activity is partly learned. Some folks unfortunately "learn" to eat to excess. But this means that they can also "learn" to control this excess.

And herein lies the key advantage of viewing a behavior as a compulsion rather than an addiction. To be a "food addict" implies that a person has a sickness or disease, and this imparts a sense of unchangeable, terminal fear. To engage in "compulsive eating" suggests that a person is experiencing a behavioral problem that he or she can learn to control, and this imparts a sense of hope for positive change.

So, What Can I Eat?

If eating is not an addiction in the true sense of the word and if abstinence is not the answer, what is an emotional/compulsive/binge eater to do after surgery? First of all, rest assured that you can still eat after weight loss surgery. It's not as if you can never eat a cookie again now that you have a gastric band, gastric sleeve or gastric bypass. What most people cannot do is eat large quantities in one sitting. Thankfully most of my patients tell me they have a reduced desire to overeat.

A common danger is *grazing*, where a person eats small quantities of food throughout the day. It's almost as if your surgery cannot detect such eating and therefore is unable to prevent it from occurring. Clearly, nobody who went through the process of having weight loss surgery has the intention of engaging in a behavior that would cause the surgery to be less effective, but it is important to realize that it can happen. Old habits die hard.

Some folks are concerned about consuming excess quantities of foods that they have heard can "cheat" the mechanism of their surgery. For example, most patients are aware that large quantities of high-calorie liquids or *meltables* like ice cream and chocolate can slip through the gastric band and decrease total weight loss. This is correct and I have seen this occur on a few occasions. However, it is important to note that reasonable quantities of ice cream, milk shakes and other high calorie liquids will not likely have that much of an impact on your overall weight loss through the years, and trying to abstain from eating such foods forever is going to be counterproductive.

And what's "reasonable" for reasonable quantities of meltables? That typically would be a few servings per month, but check with your surgeon to be sure. Five hundred calories a month from two or three servings of ice cream is unlikely to make the difference between losing 50 versus 75 pounds over the course of a year.

How Can I Avoid Binging?

What most people worry about is the possibility of *binging* on foods after surgery. The good news is that I rarely encounter a person with no history of binging before weight loss surgery who becomes a binge eater after surgery. Similarly, it is rare that someone who was not particularly fond of ice cream prior to surgery suddenly becomes an ice cream junkie afterward. If your problem before surgery had to do with controlling your intake of chicken wings, nacho chips, pretzels or pizza, then you're very unlikely to suddenly start binging on ice cream or milk shakes simply because you know you might be able to get away with it. This makes sense. When you really want nachos or pizza, would a scoop of butterscotch ice cream or a milk shake do it for you? Not likely.

Even folks who did binge on ice cream, chocolate, milk shakes and the like prior to surgery do not typically do so after surgery. Most people tell me that they generally don't feel the need to eat this way any more. Many patients can now distinguish between "head hunger" and genuine hunger. They know that their stomach is much smaller and they now feel a strong sense of fullness, which reduces or eliminates the urge to keep eating. Eating beyond this point of discomfort is now more easily identifiable as emotional eating.

But what about those who do continue to engage in self-destructive eating patterns after surgery? Is there any hope for them? Absolutely! Turn to the next chapter to find out what happens to binge eating after weight loss surgery.

10

Binge Eating After Weight Loss Surgery

DOES WEIGHT LOSS SURGERY ELIMINATE or help control binge eating? Will my gastric band, gastric bypass or gastric sleeve restrict me from eating large quantities of food? These questions are of great concern to folks with a history of binge eating who are interested in weight loss surgery. My experience working with hundreds of surgical weight loss patients suggests that weight loss surgery *initially* diminishes the desire to binge, as well as controls the amount and rate of food consumption.

However, surgery is not a foolproof cure for binge eating. I have seen several patients who resumed binge eating after weight loss surgery, many of whom regained in excess of 25 pounds in the process. Therefore, you cannot expect that weight loss surgery will "cure" binge eating. It is a behavior that may need to be addressed at some point following surgery. But before we talk about how to combat binge eating, let's define it.

What Is Binge Eating?

Binge eating or *binging* is a behavior commonly reported by people who are morbidly obese. Many patients report that a major reason they pursued weight loss surgery was a desire to control their binge eating. Let's define binge eating and dispel some of the misconceptions about its nature and how it should be treated.

The *Diagnostic and Statistical Manual of Mental Disorders* (DSM-IV-TR) defines a *binge* as follows:

1. Eating, in a discrete period of time (for example, within any two hour period), an amount of food that is definitely larger than most people would eat in a similar period of time under similar circumstances, and

2. A sense of lack of control over eating during the episode (for example, a feeling that one cannot stop eating or control what or how much they are eating).

Other common elements of binge eating include: eating much more rapidly than normal; eating until feeling uncomfortably full; eating large amounts of food when not feeling physically hungry; eating alone due to feelings of embarrassment with how much one is eating; and feelings of disgust with oneself, depression, or severe guilt after overeating. It is also common for people to make an effort to hide or conceal their binging because of embarrassment with either the manner in which the person is eating or the quantity of food being consumed. A last observation not inherent in the DSM-IV-TR definition is that binges often involve consumption of *forbidden foods*, such as chocolate, ice cream and the like. Have you ever met a person who binged on broccoli or carrots?

As with other behaviors, it's possible to identify those factors that might activate or trigger a binge episode. Commonly reported triggers of binge episodes include: feelings of tension, eating, being alone, feeling fat, breaking the rules of a diet and food cravings, among others.

Notice that the definition of a binge uses the term "most people" in identifying what is an appropriate amount of food. Most Americans eat abnormally large or supersized portions, so this criterion is slightly vague and not constant. A normal portion today would likely be considered almost obscene in 1950. To illustrate, it has been reported that the large portion of French fries in a popular hamburger chain in the 1970's is the same size as today's small portion.

Also, there is controversy over the length of time that constitutes a binge. We typically think of binging as a voracious episode of eating (think of Cookie Monster from Sesame Street). However, some people are more of what I call *grazing bingers* or simply *grazers*. These folks may not eat an abnormally large amount of food in a two-hour period, but will consume an excessive amount of food over the course of several hours or an entire day. While the quantity of food and the time frame in which it is consumed may vary, what is always present is the sense that one can't control his or her behavior.

What Binge Eating Is Not

Let's be clear about what doesn't qualify as binge eating. First, I caution you against seeing binge eating as an addiction. For many of the reasons already discussed in chapter 9, such as the dangers of feeling powerless over solving your problem, and the impossibility of abstinence, using a label like "food addiction" is misleading and counterproductive.

Second, many patients make the argument that being morbidly obese is evidence of being "out of control" of their eating. While a lack of control over eating is one criterion of binge eating disorder, simply stating or thinking that your eating is "out of control" is not sufficient to qualify for binge eating. This loose definition of lost control blurs the important distinction between having serious binges and being obese. You can be morbidly obese without having a binge eating disorder.

Third, binge eating is not evidence of an "addictive" or "compulsive" personality. In fact, much research suggests that the notion of an "addictive personality" is probably a myth—something that many people believe exists, but in reality does not. A full discussion of this controversy is beyond the scope of this book, but you'll find additional readings on the topic in appendix C.

Binge Eating Versus Emotional Eating

The clinical criteria for binge eating make no stipulation that the individual be experiencing emotional distress at the time of the binge or that some emotion triggered the binge. Oftentimes, strong emotions in the form of guilt or self-loathing follow the binge, although many binge eaters have little recollection of their emotions during a binge. Many patients describe a sense of "fogging out" or "numbing out" while they're binging. Some of the binge eaters I've counseled have shared that they often binge while in a perfectly good mood and that the only source of emotional distress they experience is the sense that they cannot control their behavior.

What binge eating and emotional eating have in common is the general sense that they represent maladaptive or undesirable eating habits. Some insist that binge eating is a subset of emotional eating, suggesting that all binge eaters are emotional eaters. But all emotional eaters are not binge eaters. What's important to understand is that they are two distinct phenomena. However, many of the tools that address emotional eating can be applied to binge eating, as well.

How Can I Reduce Binge Eating?

A first step would be to use a diary to self-monitor various aspects of your behavior. Just like you learned to monitor cravings in chapter 7 and emotions in chapter 8, you can use a diary to monitor the triggers of your binges. Use the *Cravings Diary Worksheet* in appendix B to uncover patters in your triggers. Document what you eat, when you eat, and most importantly, what you are thinking and feeling when eating. Although many people truly detest this form of self-monitoring, when it comes to binging it is without question the best tool for you to learn to identify your emotional, cognitive and behavioral triggers for binges.

Notice that I said *your* triggers. You could assume to know them, but you would be better served by tracking your behavior in as great detail as possible for a few weeks to pinpoint them more exactly. This will enable you to consider and develop alternative strategies for binge eating later on as you move toward changing your binge behavior.

Believe it or not, how you go about weighing yourself can influence whether you binge. This is a very touchy subject for most people, which is why I recommend that you weigh yourself, at most, once per week—more than that is not only unhelpful, it's harmful. Daily variations of water levels and other factors make your daily weight an almost useless number. It doesn't necessarily reflect the result of your eating behavior. Worse yet, weighing yourself each day can cause you to become obsessed with your weight and frustrated or angry with yourself. When your weight goes down, you're ecstatic. When it goes up or remains unchanged, you may become frustrated and try to speed things up by skipping meals or starving, which is very likely to trigger a binge. I often tell people that if you're weighing yourself every day, what you're really weighing is your self-esteem and self-acceptance, not your body weight. Remember this the next time you step on the scale.

Another important step in overcoming binge eating is to rid yourself of what I call *diet brain*. Diet brain involves thinking in black-and-white terms, where particular foods are categorized as being either good or bad, and self-acceptance is contingent upon whether you exhibited restraint during your most recent meal. Diet brain involves thinking of days as being good or bad based on whether you ate chocolate or whether you met your particular daily calorie goals.

Diet brain thinking is a major trigger for binging. How? Let's assume you've been dieting for several days. You step on the scale after three days and nothing has changed; in fact, maybe you've even gained a pound. When this occurs, you're likely to tell yourself something like: To hell with this, it's pointless, and I don't know why I even bother anymore! What is likely to follow is the opening of floodgates. Mass consumption of what formerly had been prohibited.

Do not strive for perfect eating. Allow yourself to accept small deviations from your plan. In fact, it is actually good to practice small deviations from your plan. Rather than thinking of some foods as "forbidden" and trying to completely avoid them (like chocolate), it would be preferable to learn to eat them in moderation. Think about it: Are you really *never* going to eat chocolate again? This is why diets fail: Because they are often built on the absolutist premise of "never," rather than the more balanced "sometimes." When your rule of "never" fails, you see yourself as a failure, which is a negative emotion that can easily prompt a binge.

My advice? Have a bite of chocolate here and there. I don't care if you think: But I've tried that before and it always leads to a binge!

The likely reason that it has always led to a binge is that you've always told yourself that you "screwed up" or were a "bad" or "weak" person for having the chocolate. Remember from chapter 9:

> Eating is *not* an addiction. It does *not* require an abstinence approach. Moderate, measured eating of risky ("forbidden") foods is the key to defeating binge eating, *not* abstinence.

It might also help if you stop calling them "forbidden" foods; I prefer the term *risky foods*, instead. Often these are the same as your *trigger foods* or *comfort foods*. You may think I am asking you to commit weight loss suicide by eating a small or moderate amount of food. I'm not. I know this approach is controversial. But in my experience, with the appropriate encouragement and support, it works.

You may notice that I seem to be suggesting that a crucial step in getting rid of diet brain is getting rid of dieting, something I cover extensively in chapter 4. Some forms of dieting are, indeed, a trigger for binge eating.

More Tips To Combat Binging

Your surgery's real strength is its ability to help control your portions. But there is more that needs to be done to lose the weight and keep it off. You'll need to incorporate the eating changes induced by your surgery into a broader lifestyle modification program. Following are a set of guidelines involving the establishment of changes in lifestyle.

1. Engage in behaviors that are incompatible with binging.

Our society has made socializing around eating the norm. It doesn't have to be that way. People can gather together around an activity that doesn't include eating at all. Adding new social behaviors to your lifestyle that don't always revolve around food and eating is the key. Skip that huge dinner with friends. Instead, try exercising with others by going for a walk or playing tennis. Discover the great outdoors through walking, biking, hiking or swimming. If none of these exercises strike a chord, find another. And try other social activities sans food as well, such as going to a street fair, museum or shopping. There's a lot to do!

With binging, eating takes center stage rather than simply being a necessary behavior to refuel the body, and you need to change that. Your new goal is to engage in activities that don't involve eating at all, or at least make it a secondary event. Rather than making a meal the central focus of your interactions with friends, substitute something more active. Make the meal a secondary activity.

2. When you eat, make eating a structured, planned activity.

I know what you're thinking: I hate structure! However, structure works! One of the most essential strategies to defeat binge eating is to eat three meals per day and perhaps one or two planned snacks. When it comes to eating: Don't wing it—plan it! Don't allow eating to be a casual, mindless behavior. Perhaps, you are one of those folks who have been battling binge eating for decades. It is possible that you may be unable to eliminate the behavior of binging entirely. It's something that you have rehearsed and performed perhaps *thousands* of times, without a structured, focused approach. You are not going to just wake up one morning and find that you no longer have the desire to eat the way you have for the past 30 years! It is going to take work and it is going to require some serious planning. Planned meals and planned snacks is a structured, focused approach that works, and is the core ingredient of virtually all treatment programs for binge eating.

3. Avoid engaging in behaviors that distract you while eating.

While you are eating, what else are you doing? Now might be a good time to check the "What am I doing? With whom?" column in your *Cravings Diary Worksheet* to see (appendix B). Sometimes these other things you do take your mind off eating, and that's not always a good thing. Turn off the television, put down the newspaper, and shut down the computer. Try to tune in to the feelings and sensations of eating to better understand and control your behavior.

92

4. Don't skip meals or go on starvation diets.

It is very important that you practice being patient with your weight loss. It will not happen overnight. With that in mind, avoid over-restriction of your food intake. Restrictions like meal skipping or starvation will not speed up the weight loss process. Rather, they are perhaps the greatest triggers for binge eating.

5. Learn new, healthy ways to cope with emotional distress.

Let's face it: You eat in response to emotion. We all do to some extent, as we learned in chapter 8. A critical step in defeating binge eating is to learn new alternative methods of coping with emotional distress that do not involve eating.

Anyone who eats for emotional reasons can tell you how silly and useless the behavior is. No matter what emotional problem confronts you, eating 20 chocolate chip cookies will not solve it! You may experience a temporary reprieve and a brief feeling of pleasure from the cookies, but the initial problem persists, and is now compounded by feelings of guilt and self-loathing for having eaten those cookies.

Consider learning relaxation strategies, taking a brief walk, listening to music or developing a social network to call upon under such circumstances. Don't be surprised if your new strategy feels awkward at first; that's to be expected. It'll take a while for you to feel comfortable without nibbling on something.

What If I Slip?

If you should have a slip of binge eating, first and foremost don't panic. And don't get down on yourself for that slip. Consider that it was bound to happen. Slip happens! Most people find it difficult to stop binge eating cold turkey, or any food for that matter. (Yes, a sense of humor is important, too!)

Having a binge is a setback, *not* a relapse. Eating one chocolate bar (a slip) is not the same as eating a pound of chocolate (a relapse). Having a binge does not put you back to square one. Telling yourself that you are a failure for having had a chocolate bar, or even two or three of them, triggers self-hatred and hopelessness. It is this self-hatred and hopelessness, not the chocolate bar, that leads you to binge even more. You can find out more about addressing slips, slides, setbacks, and relapse in chapter 12.

Need More Help With Binge Eating?

If you've had weight loss surgery and continue to struggle with binge eating, you can read more about it by consulting the resources in appendix C. If the slip keeps on slipping, and you can't seem to stop, then professional help is advisable. Binge eating is a treatable problem. Addressing it directly will help you achieve your long-term weight loss goals and significantly improve your quality of life.

Part III

Slip Slidin' Away

It's not a perfect world, and no surgery or treatment is a perfect cure. This section prepares you for lapses and relapses to eating and weight gain. In the process, we'll uncover the most prominent saboteurs of your weight loss success. Most importantly, we'll learn a new set of tools to deal with slips and setbacks, as well as strategies to prevent relapse.

11

Sabotage!

W ILL I SABOTAGE MYSELF AFTER my surgery? This is a question asked by a great number of patients before surgery. With sabotage, the common notion is that unconscious factors are going to get in the way of your efforts to lose weight or put the weight back on after you've lost it. Several daytime talk shows have featured episodes with guests who have undergone weight loss surgery and regained the weight, claiming that psychological factors were to blame. Certainly, psychological factors can interfere with weight loss or weight maintenance following surgery. However, these factors need not be unconscious and generally do not represent attempts by the patient to sabotage their efforts to succeed from surgery.

The good news is that patients who bring it up during consultation demonstrate that they are thinking ahead and want to take steps to assure the best possible outcome from surgery. These patients recognize that while surgery is a crucial tool for losing weight, it is not an automatic ticket to lasting weight loss.

A Premeditated Act?

The term *sabotage* is a rather intriguing and sexy word that conjures up images of cold war spy novels. Sabotage means to destroy or obstruct normal operations or to hinder an endeavor. By this definition, sabotage is *deliberate* and *premeditated*. Why in the world would someone who has decided to have weight loss surgery attempt to deliberately derail efforts to lose weight? After all of the years of suffering with obesity and struggling with diet after diet, what could possibly motivate an effort to make the surgery fail?

There are a number of factors at work and some are easier to identify and change than others. Most people are *not* trying to interfere with their surgery's efforts to enable weight loss. What is probably happening is that old habits and unresolved issues that may have contributed to the original weight gain before surgery are still in play. As we've seen with craving (chapter 7), emotional eating (chapter 8), and binging (chapter 10), old habits die hard.

In sum, although it makes for great superficial talk show fodder, the phenomenon known as "sabotage" is misleading and inappropriate. As with all efforts designed to garner your attention and get you to tune in, it preys on your natural fear that weight loss surgery might not succeed. Plus it creates undue anxiety, suggesting that you deliberately did something wrong.

Defeating the Saboteurs

Sabotage can be a usable concept if we remove premeditation and the notion that it's deliberate. When sabotage refers to unconscious motivations or factors outside of our awareness that complicate the road to sustained weight loss, we can even become empowered as we devise battle strategies to defeat these saboteurs!

A good start would be to take the time to recall what interfered with your ability to lose or maintain weight loss on those diets you tried in the past. Do this actively: Make a list and write it down. Perfect for this purpose is the *Diet Trials Worksheet* in appendix B, which asks you to delve into your past and recollect recent diets. This worksheet compels you to examine what prompted you to start the diet, stop the diet, and record what happened. When you begin to look systematically at the circumstances surrounding each diet, a clear picture of your saboteurs will begin to emerge. Consider the following example:

> Last New Year's Day you began a diet that lasted about six weeks. You were prompted to begin the diet because you thought the start of a new year was a good enough reason as any. As part of your attempt to lose weight, you also joined a health club and attended twice a week. Impressive!
>
> But once February arrived, your plan began to crumble. You thought that because you were exercising you didn't have to diet as much anymore. As you began eating more, those four pounds that you worked so hard to lose up to this point quickly reappeared.
>
> You put in all this work exercising while trying to diet, and you felt dejected about winding up back where you started. The futile nature of the whole endeavor caused you to eat even more, and by the end of February you gained another nine pounds.

So there were a few saboteurs in this scenario. Your reason to start the diet was arbitrary (the New Year), so it held no motivational imperative. And although joining the health club was truly laudable, exercise alone will not help you maintain weight loss. You've got to also decrease your food intake. When the weight returned, you gave up and dealt with the futile exercise through emotional eating.

Without question on many occasions the saboteurs are simply the problems that we *all* encounter when trying to lose weight: the feelings of hunger, deprivation, irritability, and the monotony of most diets. These problems are quite common and very straightforward—no hidden saboteurs here. As you know from chapter 4, dieting is inherently unpleasant and therefore most people have trouble sticking with diets for more than a few days or weeks. This is probably the single greatest reason people struggle to remain on diets for the long haul. It is very difficult to deprive yourself and be hungry, possibly irritable and compliant for years upon years.

Other times, however, the reasons for relapse may have been more complex. Was your busy lifestyle the problem? I'm sure it was to some degree. Were others in your household not supportive? Was your commitment to the diet and your level of planning adequate?

Were there emotional factors involved? Hmm, now we're getting warmer! Was there any discomfort associated with becoming thinner? Did you find yourself experiencing any unpleasant feelings as the weight came off? Did others treat you differently when you were thinner? Was their treatment uncomfortable to you in any way? Oh! Very interesting questions!

Identifying less obvious patterns in the causes of relapse from weight loss efforts in the past may provide you with valuable clues to areas that need to be addressed to ensure that they do not disrupt your weight loss efforts following weight loss surgery. To find these issues, you have to dig deeper, asking yourself some difficult questions and being very honest with the answers. These are the saboteurs that are hiding in the darkness, outside of your immediate awareness. What were the feelings and experiences you had when you were thinner that you may not readily want to acknowledge or discuss?

Even if you do not feel particularly vulnerable to saboteurs and cannot immediately recognize any emotional hot spots on the horizon or in your past, it would still be worthwhile to ask yourself some of these questions. Ask any surgical weight loss patient and she will tell you that she's learned ways to "eat around" her surgery if she is so motivated. Unless you make the effort to address these potential saboteurs, you could very well jeopardize your surgery. I want to be very clear about this:

> No matter which surgery you have, if you do not address the emotional factors that have contributed to your eating or address issues that arise as a result of your weight loss through surgery, your weight loss may be short lived.

Is Being Thin Enough?

Many overweight people fantasize about thinness. Although some express an understanding that being thinner doesn't make everything better, there is this general notion that most things would be better. At the very least they understand that the world seems better suited to those of a normal weight. Clothes are easier to buy and look better. Thinner people generally get treated better than overweight people. This is all generally true. But not everything in everyone's life improves as a result of becoming thinner. In fact, at least for a little while, it often gets worse. In my experience, the folks who regain weight for emotional reasons often regain because they resume eating to cope with some of the hardships that ensue from being *thinner*! Don't believe me? Read on!

At first, it's wonderful. The pounds begin to melt off, everyone is a cheerleader and the news is all good. However, I've seen a number of patients whose weight loss prematurely reached a plateau several months or a year or so after surgery. They knew that emotional factors were getting in the way, even though they wanted to believe that simply adjusting their gastric band, hitting the gym, or making some dietary changes would work things out.

A significant number of patients who encountered emotional difficulties related to being thinner following surgery had *some* suspicion that these difficulties might emerge. In fact, it was not unusual for some patients to bring up these concerns during the pre-surgical evaluation. For these folks, the saboteur is hardly a mysterious agent that lurks in the darkness. Rather, it's a problem hibernating in a cave of obesity. When the weight melts away, the problem quickly comes out of hibernation. They are just uncomfortable being thinner.

Some of the more common saboteurs of weight loss that my patients report include:

- ✓ Receiving too much attention from others—becoming "visible."
- ✓ Fears of intimacy and physical or sexual relationships.
- ✓ Fears of increased expectations from yourself and others.
- ✓ Being unable to let go of self-hatred and feeling like a failure.
- ✓ Jealousy from others and changes in the dynamics of personal relationships.
- ✓ Fears of having to make major life changes to achieve your goals.

Notice that most of these concerns relate to fear or anxiety. Also notice that much of the anxiety relates to the relationships we have with others. So it seems that most of the post-surgical saboteurs are social and scary! Let's look at each of these more closely as we develop our battle plan to overcome the saboteurs.

I'm No Longer Invisible

This is one of the most common sources of discomfort following surgery. I am astounded by how many patients refer to feelings of being *invisible* in their obesity and how exposed they feel by being thinner. Prior to surgery these patients tell me that despite their size, they have felt invisible for much of their lives. It's as if others didn't notice them, or more likely chose not to acknowledge their presence.

The sad truth is that the world doesn't like fat people. (Pardon me for using the F-word, but it better conveys the feelings these folks have than the politically correct ways of saying fat, such as heavy or overweight.) Many people try not to look at fat people. They don't hold the door open for them. They avoid eye contact with fat people and don't give the friendly smile when incidental eye contact occurs. Fat people feel oddly and sadly invisible.

It may be difficult to imagine that nobody notices you when you're 100 pounds overweight. Of course it's not that they don't notice you—they are *choosing* to ignore you. If *others* don't acknowledge your existence, it's not that hard to understand how *you* could begin to feel that they may not be able to see you. You are invisible. But then you have the surgery and begin to lose weight. Suddenly, you are on everyone's radar. Eye contact is made, smiles are exchanged, as you begin to hear those formerly elusive hellos. All of a sudden, you're in clear view—high definition, no less!

Fear of Intimacy

For many, the attention received after losing a lot of weight is entirely welcome and enjoyable. However, if you've been emotionally, physically or sexually abused, it is understandable that suddenly becoming visible to others could trigger a good bit of anxiety. Imagine a formerly obese woman who had been sexually abused years ago who became thin again for the first time in over 20 years. She is becoming increasingly aware of the wandering eyes of male strangers at her thinner body and it's making her uncomfortable. Is it not easy to see how she might resort to her age-old coping mechanism of eating to help ease her anxiety? Of course she doesn't want to, but if she hasn't developed any new methods of addressing her anxiety, she will likely head straight for the refrigerator. In the short run, her eating will minimize her distress. In the long run, the resulting weight gain will make her feel less attractive, and therefore less vulnerable and less threatened by others.

Even in the absence of a past history of sexual abuse, the sudden attention from others and the resulting visibility could create anxiety and a feeling of awkwardness. Now that others are interacting with you, you feel as if you have to pass muster in their eyes. All the world is a stage and everyone is watching. This could lead you to eat to seek comfort from the anxiety of all the attention.

It may seem ironically ridiculous that you would engage in the very same eating behavior that got you into trouble in the past. But if that's all you know, that's what you do. As I've said before, humans are abysmal at tolerating emotional discomfort. We all have developed strategies to help us cope with unpleasant emotions, and we use these strategies almost reflexively when life gets uncomfortable. These old strategies lurk in the shadows like saboteurs, waiting to jump into action. Unless we develop new strategies, the old ones will persist and prevail.

Unreasonable Expectations

Fears of increased expectations from others and greater responsibility for your own success are also quite common. There is absolutely no truth to the widely held belief that overweight people are lazy or unmotivated. In fact, the opposite may be true. You will never find a group of people more motivated to accomplish a goal than obese people trying to lose weight. However, if many people in your world seem to believe that you are lazy and unmotivated, you may have learned to believe it yourself, as unreasonable expectations lead to a dangerous *self-fulfilling prophecy*.

The laziness label may not be true for losing weight because it's something you've probably tried a number of times. However, it is possible that you didn't demand as much from yourself in other areas of your life, or that others made excuses for you because of your weight. Maybe you believed that some of your goals were simply not achievable because you were overweight.

It's understandable that as you lose weight following surgery, both you and others may raise the bar on your expectations for achievement. If your weight was a primary reason that you avoided pursuing the things you want in life, it makes sense that you would be anxious now that your weight is decreasing. Questions will arise. Can I do it? Was it just the weight holding me back? What if I fail in pursuit of this goal? These questions give rise to anxiety, which again could cause someone to revert back to eating as a method of coping, and eventually to weight regain.

Anger

Many patients who have successfully lost weight share that they are now angry with themselves for having let themselves "get so fat" and for not doing anything about it for so long. Ah—if hindsight was only 20/20! Many patients I have counseled prior to surgery report poor self-esteem, associating their total self-worth with the number on the scale or the waist size of their pants. Many have been brainwashed into believing that if they just had a little more willpower, their obesity never would have occurred.

But now that they're thinner and have gone through an extraordinary struggle to address their archnemesis obesity, they're back to believing the nonsense they had fought so hard to reject in the first place! Of course, such thoughts are nonsense, as we know from chapters 3, 4, and 5. Science has all but confirmed that obesity is a biological phenomenon, greatly influenced by genetic, behavioral, social, and societal factors. Willpower is not the problem. While your behavior did have something to do with it, blaming yourself for your inability to resolve your weight problem prior to surgery is just silly.

Now that you made the brave decision to have surgery, it's important that you applaud yourself for having done so! It's important that you treat yourself with dignity and respect and to *insist* that others treat you with dignity and respect. There is simply no benefit to berating yourself for having been obese. This kind of thinking will result in nothing productive and unfortunately could lead to unpleasant feelings and unhealthy emotional eating.

Jealousy

Unfortunately, there is a real chance that at least one friend or family member will be jealous of your weight loss. The dynamics of a few of your relationships may change. While you are achieving your weight loss goals, those around you who are struggling to do the same are left with two options: Applaud you for your success or diminish your accomplishment. The latter is sometimes the path others choose. At least one person is going to suggest that you "cheated" by losing weight through having surgery instead of the assumedly correct method of diet and exercise. Of course, this is total bull. The jealousy of others is the saboteur.

Don't give in to your first impulse of anger. Instead, talk it over with the jealous person. If it's truly a good relationship, it will endure. If the other person happens to be morbidly obese, it may be that she is frustrated with her own struggle and is not yet ready to consider surgery for herself. You could be very helpful to this person.

Sadly, you may need to say goodbye to some who you thought were close friends but who now are no longer. Ending long-time relationships is very difficult. A number of patients have found that their social life was much more complicated now that they were thinner. I have known more than one patient who chose to put weight back on to make her social life work better. A particular patient's friends remained overweight and seemed to feel that she could no longer relate to them. They stopped going out to eat with her and stopped sharing their diet war stories with her, thinking she wouldn't understand. This was probably not true, but they acted differently toward her and the relationships had changed. She opted to open her gastric band, which enabled her to eat more and put some of the weight back on. This was a purposeful decision, although probably not one in her best interest.

Fear of Change

I remember contributing to an article in a magazine about how weight loss surgery causes major changes in people's lives. Unfortunately, the way the article was written it suggested that weight loss surgery was almost dangerous in terms of the unexpected changes that it could produce. In the story, a woman lost over 100 pounds and then promptly ended her marriage, which turned her whole life upside down. What the coauthor of the article failed to mention was that she entered the marriage knowing that she wasn't really in love with her husband in the first place. In other words, she settled for him because of her weight. She didn't think she could do any better. In this case, the surgery didn't cause major changes in her life. Rather, it gave her the opportunity to make some major changes. For many, this is exactly why they choose to have surgery: to have the opportunity to take action on things they've put on hold. For many obese individuals, much of their life has been on hold.

This story highlights how important it is for you to be honest with yourself and ask yourself some tough questions before having surgery. What will change when I'm thinner? Am I ready for these changes? The woman in the magazine story is very much like many folks I've counseled after the surgery. How will losing weight affect your marriage or your relationship with your partner? How will your weight loss affect them? Just as importantly, how will it affect you? Honest answers to these questions will increase your chances of weight loss success.

Let's delve deeper: What is the current state of your relationship? What would change if you were thinner? Did your weight have a major impact on the person you chose to be with? Has the weight significantly altered the relationship to the point that you want out of the relationship?

I have worked with a number of people who have had extramarital affairs following surgery. Many of them were surprised at their behavior and some were ashamed. Almost all were unsure of how it happened. It was likely that opportunities that had not been there for years suddenly became available, and they had little experience managing those opportunities and setting appropriate boundaries. With new social opportunities, some have decided to indulge, and this can upset the apple cart at home.

Clearly I am not suggesting that staying in an unsatisfying relationship is preferable. I'm also not condoning having extramarital affairs. What I am suggesting is that you take a very close and careful look at the state of your intimate relationships and try to anticipate how you want things to go. You need to do this so that you won't be surprised by how things turn out. Some patients are quite frank as to their intentions, and for these folks life changes don't come as a surprise—they are part of the plan.

One woman who had become thinner after weight loss surgery was quite explicit. In no uncertain terms, she said, "I don't really enjoy my marriage anymore and haven't for some time. I was in my marriage because I didn't think anybody else would have me at my old weight. With my new weight, I feel different, and I am going to test the waters." This woman separated from her husband and started dating again, and eventually found a new life partner.

Thus far, I've focused primarily on how being thinner can affect social and intimate relationships, and you'll learn even more about dealing with relationships in part IV of this book. However, the same principles apply to one's career. Many have shared their fears of interviewing for jobs when obese, believing they would be all but laughed out of the door. But after losing weight, the excuse of weight discrimination dissolves. Now you have to ask yourself new questions: Are you happy with your job? If not, what you are going to do about it?

Being overweight provides an almost believable excuse to leave things as they are, however unsatisfying they may be. By losing weight you will open up the doors to many new and often exciting possibilities. But remember to be mindful of saboteurs on the other side that might keep you from moving forward in a healthy and successful manner. I'm certainly not advocating that you turn away from opening the door. I'm just strongly encouraging you to prepare a bit before turning that knob.

12

Slips, Slides, Setbacks and Relapse

YOU'VE STUMBLED UPON A LOOPHOLE in the weight loss surgery universe. Maybe you ate something that you think you shouldn't have eaten. Or maybe you were able to eat something that you thought your surgery would prevent you from eating. This was the moment that you feared and you're probably quite concerned about what happens next. If you're like many people at this juncture, you're worried that this slip represents a tiny piece of loose string that will allow the entire ball of yarn to unwind and for the weight to gradually come back. This is one of the most common concerns expressed by my patients. But don't panic—it was bound to happen. In fact, it may actually be a good thing.

You've certainly been here before. We can all remember times when we were dieting with great success, and for a brief while it felt as if we were on autopilot—that we finally won the war and were going to lose the weight *and* keep it off. Then a funny thing happened on the way to wearing slim cut jeans. A single high calorie day occurred that turned into two days, then three, and before you knew it, a week. And then seemingly overnight, every last pound you lost, and maybe a few more, came back.

Here's the good news: It doesn't have to happen again. Having a slip is not the end of the world. In fact, it doesn't need to amount to more than a blip on the radar. How you think about the slip and what you do in response to it is crucial to your weight loss success.

Recognizing Slippery Territory

Let's distinguish between a slip, a slide, a setback, and a relapse. Understanding these distinctions is essential. Think of a *slip*, sometimes called a *lapse*, as being an "oops," something that began without you even being aware of it. This is how *mindless eating* begins (first covered in chapters 7 and 8), though it need not continue if you can catch yourself. You ate something you believe you shouldn't have—a chocolate bar, a bag of chips, a slice of pizza. Maybe you ate two cookies instead of one. Perhaps you even had a very small binge. Regardless, a single episode of eating is rarely more than a slip.

A *slide* is a planned slip. You *decided* to have a slip. You decided to eat a cookie or some chips rather than allowing an "oops" to unknowingly unfold. The food wasn't just sitting there and "oops" you had a few. Instead you walked into the kitchen from the living room with the intention of having a few potato chips.

A *setback* is a more prolonged slip or slide. It's not just an off-moment, but perhaps an off-day or an off-few-days. You're eating in a manner that's not with the program, and momentum is building in the wrong direction. When people go off their diet over the weekend or on a vacation we could call this a setback.

A *relapse* is a full return to a previous, problematic state, not only in terms of your eating behavior, but of your mindset, as well. During a relapse, you're eating in a manner that is more consistent with the old days than the time since you've had surgery. A good example of a relapse is what happens to many folks when they return from vacation. You have the full intention of getting back to your planned healthy eating, but the setback that occurred during the vacation now has momentum on its side. And on the Monday after vacation, your return to healthy eating doesn't stand a chance. You're eating like you did before the diet. What's even more problematic is that during a relapse, your mindset has changed, as well. You start to experience feelings of hopelessness and self-loathing. Most people don't think of a relapse as an "oops." They start thinking: Why do I even bother? It's pointless! What's wrong with me that I can never stick to healthy eating? I'm a failure.

As you try to make sense of all these distinctions, it's important to recognize one very important thing:

Slip happens!

It is not possible to go through your entire life without giving in to temptation. In fact, it is common to have numerous slips. Could you imagine living the next 30 years without a single taste of chocolate? Would you even want to? Viewed in a certain manner, slips can actually be both enjoyable and valuable. And this is why it's okay to take some *slide rides* (planned slips) every once in a while. Many people look forward to Thanksgiving and it's not for their love of pilgrims. Thanksgiving could aptly be called National Eating Day. Enjoying all of the fruits (and apple pies!) of Thanksgiving is the equivalent of a slide. Surely nobody says that Thanksgiving has to be an all out eating frenzy. But most of us consume a bit more than usual on turkey day. If it ends with the final piece of pie, then no harm is done.

There's another benefit to having a slide and it could be one of the keys to true success. Learning to eat highly rewarding foods (sometimes called *risky foods, trigger foods, forbidden foods,* or *comfort foods*) in a controlled manner shows that you're in charge of your eating and that you've truly changed. This we already discussed in chapter 10. Dieting promotes absolutist thinking—black-and-white, pass or fail. It does *not* teach you how to eat properly. It teaches your how to either avoid certain foods or overeat them. When we're on diets we restrict, and when we're off diets we binge. Neither involves healthy eating.

Think about your long history of failed diets for a moment. Isn't it self-control that you've been after? Haven't you always truly wished that you could just have a bite and end it at that? Learning to slip and immediately get on track again is just that skill. And every once in a while, you'll be able to take safe slide rides. It is critical for your long-term success that you learn to do this. I understand you're skeptical and scared. You're thinking that you've been lulled into this delusion of portion control before and that it has always resulted in total weight regain. But it doesn't have to be that way. With a few slip-management tools in your belt, you'll be able to reverse those old patterns.

As you learn how to manage slips, you need to *confront* food head on, not *avoid* it. This may be different from what you've learned before. Diets that promote abstinence (Overeaters Anonymous, among others) urge that you avoid highly rewarding foods, particularly those with sugar. But let's get real, here: You *know* that you are almost certainly going to have something with sugar at some point. Life is long—slips happen! Instead of avoiding, it's better to learn how to negotiate risky foods by learning skills that will address your slips. If you don't learn new skills, the only thing you'll have are feelings of guilt and shame for having eaten something you believe you should not, and feelings of hopelessness for having screwed up yet again. This is not good. It's better to learn how to eat risky foods like sugar in a controlled manner, and to think of sugar consumption as slips or slides instead of a failure of will. And it's better to learn new skills to keep slips and slides from becoming setbacks and relapses.

Stoppin' the Slippin' and Slidin'

The real danger occurs when we allow a slip or a slide to become a setback, and maybe even a relapse. This often happens when we endorse irrational beliefs about our eating behavior, when we tell ourselves distorted messages that give us permission to fall off the bandwagon. When we move toward relapse, not only is our eating changing, but our thoughts start changing, as well.

This is one of those points in the book where I'm going to say something important. Ready? Here we go: How you think is everything. In case you zoned out for a moment, let me repeat that:

How you think is everything.

This phrase is not a saying lifted from a motivational poster. What you think invariably determines what you do. It is crucial you recognize that through your thoughts *you* determine what path you're going to choose. The fact that you ate a piece of chocolate is irrelevant. Those 200 calories are inconsequential. Rather, what you tell yourself about what has just happened is the important thing. Let's illustrate this through an example:

> Imagine that it's Friday afternoon, and you're giving your child an after school snack. In the process of putting a few cookies on the plate, an extra cookie slips out of the package. Rather than putting it back, you eat it. Having enjoyed the cookie, you decide to have two more. Uh oh! You start to experience feelings of guilt, and somewhere inside you hear that voice saying, I ruined my day.
>
> A few hours later it's dinner time. Recalling that you had a few cookies earlier in the day, you decide to indulge a bit further and order tons of Chinese food, promising yourself that you'll get back on track in the morning. The next morning, you feel guilty for yesterday's indulgence and although you want to get back on track, you are reminded that you have a party to go to that evening. So you decide to let the reigns go further by telling yourself that you've already pretty much screwed up both Friday and Saturday, so why not simply let your eating go for the entire weekend and return to the program Monday morning.
>
> But come Monday, you notice that you're craving those rich foods a little more and it's harder to reinstitute that disciplined eating you found easier just a few days before. You step on the scale and see that you gained a pound. You start to feel depressed and angry with yourself and tell yourself that it's happening all over again. You start wondering if it's even worth continuing.

What's important to recognize in the example above is that you made a number of choices based upon what you were thinking, and what you were thinking guided your behavior every step of the way. There were several distinct forks in the road. Each fork was an independent decision, a choice. With each decision that took you in the wrong direction, it got much harder for you to make the next decision and turn in the right direction. It's a bit like stepping into quicksand: You tell yourself that you can turn around and walk out of it at any moment until suddenly you're in too deep to move your legs.

Let's go back and review this downward spiral, and explore how to prevent it. First we'll dissect the example by taking an honest look at what might be called your "old thinking," or what went wrong. Then we'll consider some "new thinking," or how you could have handled the situation differently.

Old thinking.

What happened when you ate that first cookie was a slip. Now you know from what I said earlier that *slips happen*, so it should have been no big deal. But it became a huge deal because your immediate thought was that it ruined your day. That belief was irrational. One cookie cannot ruin a day. But it is precisely this first fatalistic belief that set the stage for having Chinese food later in the day, a setback. By believing that you ruined you day, you told yourself that nothing you could do for the rest of the day mattered—it was hopeless; you had already failed. With this "it doesn't matter" belief in mind, you actually gave yourself permission to keep eating!

By Saturday morning, you were gaining momentum in the wrong direction. That morning, you could have ended the setback by limiting the slip to Friday. Remember, you originally thought you ruined only one day. But instead, you allowed your thoughts to lump the episode into an entire weekend. That smaller irrational belief quickly blossomed into something much worse! Not only was a single day ruined; the entire weekend was lost! Giving up on the entire weekend put you well on the way to relapse.

So in this context of growing irrational thoughts, it wasn't unreasonable for you to concede defeat until Monday, when somehow magically you thought the slate would be wiped clean. But getting things moving in the right direction again on Monday would become infinitely more difficult. On Monday, your cravings, appetite and irrational beliefs would continue to snowball. Whatever small gains you made before that first cookie on Friday now felt distant and lost, and it was hard for you to feel nothing but utterly defeated.

It may sound crazy when I dissect your thoughts this way, but this is precisely how an irrational brain thinks. This type of groundless thinking is what I called *diet brain*, discussed more fully in chapter 10. Recall that diet brain occurs when we endorse black-and-white, rigid thinking about food and eating. Diet brain puts you on a clear trajectory for relapse.

New thinking.

Let's examine what you could have done differently. After eating a few cookies, you could have told yourself that it's perfectly normal to have a few cookies once in a while. Instead of proclaiming your day a total loss, you instead could have told yourself that you eating those 100 calories of cookies that day was really not a big deal. Why? Consider that categorizing your eating by days is a behavior that remains from your old dieting attempts. Food logs, diet minders and calorie counters have to be structured around some period of time, so days seem perfectly appropriate. But if you think about it, your body doesn't count calories by days; it counts them overall. At midnight, the previous day's calories just don't disappear. You actually lose weight by controlling your calories throughout a lifetime, not in arbitrarily set chunks of 24 hours. Therefore, it's impossible to ruin an entire day by eating 100 calories of cookies. All you really did was have a high number of calories in five minutes time. So what? When you eat dinner, you probably eat around 750 calories in 30 minutes. However, you never find this upsetting because *you tell yourself* that eating 750 calories at dinner time is acceptable and normal. So you see, it all comes down to what you tell yourself—what you think.

In addition to not getting down on yourself for those 100 calories, you might try to identify what allowed the slip to occur. Try to figure out why you snuck that first cookie. Was it because it just looked so scrumptious? How is that bad? (It's not.) Why was the cookie so hard to resist? You could even take out your *Cravings Diary Worksheet* (appendix B) and write down what happened, along with your thoughts and feelings. You might uncover that you were in a bad mood at the moment, or that you were feeling particularly busy and stressed that day. If so, good—you've learned a bit more about the kind of triggers that can cause a slip for you. Or if you can't come up with a good answer, remember not to sweat it. It wasn't a big deal anyway, and you shouldn't let your mind convince you otherwise.

By rejecting thoughts of failure, you can avoid belittling herself and steer clear of strong guilt. Remember, unhealthy feelings of guilt and self-deprecation were the true emotional triggers for ordering that Chinese food, not the consumption of a few cookies.

What If I Relapse?

After a setback, it's time to reassess. What is happening and why? Why is my eating behavior moving backwards? What are the triggers? Determine if you are explicitly eating foods that you know can defeat your surgery. For example, are you eating foods that can slip through the gastric band, such as ice cream, or are you eating foods in combination with liquids to help them slide down? In either case, recognize that you are doing something to enable yourself to eat. This is not simply a lapse of willpower, but rather an active effort on your part to get food down. Why are you doing this?

A relapse is a prolonged setback. There is no set definition of how long a setback must go on before it is considered a relapse. A relapse is best defined by your mentality, more specifically the catastrophic nature of your thoughts. A relapse is basically: I quit...why bother? On the bright side, a relapse doesn't necessarily return you back to square one, because you probably have not regained all of your weight and still have much success to show for your past efforts. However, during a relapse there is probably some part of you that recognizes you are on a bad path. And you feel more vulnerable than you would like to admit.

A relapse is a serious event, and you need to take some very important steps to put yourself back on the right track to healthy eating. If you cannot do it alone, it's important to seek outside help. Your first call should be to a psychologist or other counselor who could be very helpful in keeping you focused, as well as help you determine what factors may have contributed to getting off track. If support groups are available, this would be a good time to make contact. You should try to reach out to others whom you believe could help you with your relapse. For example, tell friends and family that you need to regroup and would like their support. If you have a gastric band, you may want to contact your surgeon about possibly tightening the band. A consultation with the nutritionist might be a good idea, as well.

It's very important to remember that it is *never too late* to turn things around. The first step and the most essential step is to gather your thoughts, acknowledge what is happening and adopt the mindset that you can get things back on the right track. Make every effort to avoid thinking in ways that promote hopelessness (It's never going to be any different), helplessness (I can't do anything about it) and self-hatred (I'm such a failure; there must be something wrong with me). These thoughts are irrational, incorrect and worst of all lead to unpleasant feelings that likely promote the very behavior you're trying to change: eating!

13

Keeping It Off: Making Changes That Last

NOW THAT YOU'VE HAD WEIGHT loss surgery, one of your top priorities should be to keep the weight off for good. Concern about weight regain creates a tremendous amount of anxiety for many patients. As you know from chapter 4, the overwhelming majority of people who lose weight through diets, exercise programs, medications and other methods will see most or all of it return within a year or two. Aside from surgery, there is no method that has reliably demonstrated effective long-term weight loss for people more than 100 pounds overweight. So obviously, trepidation about weight regain is warranted. By being concerned about regaining weight, you'll be motivated to learn the skills necessary to ensure it doesn't happen.

Most surgeons and weight loss surgery professionals agree that the first year after surgery is critical in modifying your behavior. It is advisable to start making such changes as soon as possible, even prior to surgery, to try to improve your eating habits and your relationship with food. There are two sets of behavior changes that you'll need to make. First are the dietary behavior changes that are necessary based on your specific surgery. Second are the more elusive lifestyle behavior changes. We'll explore both in this chapter.

Dietary Behavior Changes

Many of the behavior changes required after weight loss surgery focus on *dietary behavior changes*, involving how and what you can and cannot eat. These are the changes you must absolutely make for your surgery to help you lose weight and for you to avoid some of the adverse consequences of weight loss surgery.

For example, if you had a gastric bypass, you've likely been warned about *dumping syndrome* (nausea, vomiting, bloating, cramping, diarrhea, dizziness, fatigue and other symptoms from small intestine expansion after consuming certain foods). You have been advised to be cautious about consuming sweets. It's likely that you've also been advised to focus on consuming adequate amounts of protein and to make sure you take an assortment of daily supplements.

If you've had gastric band surgery, you were likely informed about the perils of eating steak, doughy bread, shrimp and other foods that can get stuck in the band. You may also have been advised to stay away from high-calorie liquid sweets or *meltables* like chocolate, ice cream and milk shakes that easily slide through the band and prevent weight loss or allow for weight regain. There are other important dietary changes that go along with each surgery, and your dietician or nutritionist is a valuable resource for help on these matters.

The surgeries often force certain behavior changes, and make noncompliance with other changes quite unpleasant. For example, the discomfort and regurgitating that often occur when a gastric band patient eats a bagel generally does a good job of curtailing that behavior. Although it isn't the preferred method of learning, it is effective. Similarly, dumping syndrome often helps bypass patients avoid sweets due to its unpleasant effects.

Lifestyle Behavior Changes

Other than those dietary behavior changes discussed above, most of the changes necessary for long-term success with weight loss surgery are optional and therefore a bit more challenging. Learning to make behavior changes that you don't have to make, but should make, is essential for keeping the weight off in the long haul. These *lifestyle behavior changes* involve those thoughts, feelings, and behaviors that have typically triggered your eating in the past.

During the first several months after surgery, the anatomical changes produced by your surgery will be a good ally in your battle against weight gain. Your stomach is smaller so you're probably getting full much sooner. You probably will find that you don't get hungry like you used to, or that you're overall interest in food isn't what it used to be. Eating at this stage can actually feel difficult in many ways, so at first it might seem almost impossible *not* to lose weight. But don't be lulled into believing that you're invincible. You still need to do the work of making permanent behavioral and emotional changes when it comes to food and eating.

Thankfully, many of the postoperative patients that I've met indicate that their desire to eat has greatly diminished, and that turning the other cheek when the dessert cart arrives becomes much easier after surgery. Unfortunately, some of the folks who felt "cured" of their emotional and other eating issues during the first few months or years after surgery found those same issues gradually cropping up a bit further down the road. The band or bypass are always helping, but it's possible to get used to their effect and unwittingly learn to eat your way around them.

Like with anything that's off to a good start, the first year or so after surgery is a *honeymoon phase*. During this phase, weight loss may seem relatively easy. You may be lulled into believing that your weight problem has been fixed and feel like you're destined for eternal thinness. It's important to avoid this mindset. Once again, I encourage you to begin making changes in your eating behaviors immediately after surgery, rather than waiting until it becomes urgent to do so.

During the first year after weight loss surgery, there is a perfect window of opportunity to make these changes. Your surgery is new and its positive effects will be robust in helping you achieve success. It's the right time to solidify your new relationship with food and eating. If you are to truly win this battle with weight, you can't just wing it. Shall we begin?

Know Your Enemy

Before you develop a strategy to minimize weight gain after surgery, you'll find it helpful to identify some of your past enemies. Throughout the book, we've already discussed a number of behaviors that have hindered your battle with obesity in the past. These same behaviors haven't departed just because you've had surgery. They were probably hiding during the honeymoon phase right after surgery, so if you don't remain vigilant they'll resurface when you least expect it.

Eating on autopilot, or *mindless eating* (chapters 7, 8 and 12) can easily disrupt your recovery. Consuming food in an unhealthy way in response to negative feelings, or *emotional eating* (chapter 8), is a major trigger of setbacks and relapse. And if you were prone to *binge eating* (chapter 5) prior to surgery, now is the time to be especially watchful for its recurrence. All three of these unhealthy behaviors must remain on your radar. Now would be an excellent time to revisit earlier chapters to remind yourself how to change those behaviors.

Taking Stock of Your Arsenal

Think back to the days before surgery when you made all those efforts to lose weight on one diet after another. You had a whole arsenal of tools, tactic, techniques, and tricks to help you along the way. Now it's time to put some of that good information to use. The simpler quickie diets likely focused on some form of mathematics: calories, fat grams, portion sizes, and so on. Because their primary focus was numbers, success from these diets didn't last very long, if at all.

The better diets and weight management programs not only focus on *what* to eat, but *how* to eat. Such programs try to make permanent modifications in your lifestyle and behavior beyond simply calculating the number of calories or carbohydrates in your food. Although these programs may not have fared better for you than the quickie diets, the behavior changes they recommended were important and could come in handy now that you've had surgery.

Many patients tell me that after stopping specific diets, they've continued to maintain some of the behavior changes from these diets, even though the weight came back. Some still write down what they eat. Others have moderated their portion sizes. Still others recognize that they are now making better food choices, like switching to lower fat milk or using less butter on their bread. Keep doing whatever techniques you have found to be helpful. They remain an important part of your behavior change repertoire.

Now that you've had surgery, you have the opportunity to combine these older effective techniques with some new behavior changes, and then put all of your knowledge and skills together with the power of surgery to finally get the weight off and keep it off. Combining these behavior changes with the positive effects of surgery is a potent blend. Next, let's learn about some new behavior changes that you can try.

Adding New Techniques To Your Arsenal

There are two basic types of behavior changes you can make: One is to avoid, and the other is to alter. The basic premise of *avoidance* with regard to food is to stay away from it! By avoiding food, eating is less tempting and you'll be better able to prevent setbacks. However, it's important to realize that you cannot rely solely on avoiding food as a means of changing your eating behavior. Furthermore, it's dangerous to dogmatically employ *abstinence* with food, as we saw in chapter 9. There would be a stiff price to pay to avoid every situation that involves food or eating. You would be unable to go to the movies where they sell popcorn. You could not go to a baseball game. You could not attend a wedding.

Alteration strategies are designed to change how you behave in the presence of food without avoiding food completely. How am I going to eat differently in this situation? What am I going to do in this situation rather than eat? These are the kinds of questions addressed by alteration. Given that the absolute avoidance of food is impossible, alteration strategies are probably going to be the most important for you to learn.

Below are a number of eating and lifestyle changes that involve avoidance or alteration. I strongly recommend that you try as many of these behavioral changes as possible.

A. Preparing Your Home

1. Don't bring it in the house (avoidance).

This is pretty straightforward stuff and I'm sure you've tried to keep food out of your house before. Now do it for life! It's funny how we deceive ourselves in the supermarket. It's time for let's make a deal! See if you can recall saying some of this nonsense to yourself in the past:

> I'll have some cookies today and on Tuesday and Wednesday I'll do 50 minutes on the treadmill. Yeah, sure you will.

> I'll buy the cookies, but I'll eat just one or two a day over the next few weeks. Okay, whatever you say.

Stop kidding yourself! Don't make promises that you've never been able to keep in the past. What makes you think you'll fare better this time? Take an *honest* look back at your history and decide if what you say you want to do is realistic and reasonable.

Instead, buy a serving size of what you want when you want it, and don't have it in the house at other times. You can't eat what isn't there! Having to go to the store to buy a treat is more inconvenient and so decreases the chance that you'll ever eat the food. Having it in the house makes it almost impossible to resist.

And while we're at it, stop using your children as an excuse. For one thing, they don't need the food, either. Second, consider that if they absolutely, positively *had* to have it, you could always run a quick errand and get it for them. If you kept only healthier snacks around, believe me: They would learn to eat and enjoy them just fine.

The occasional indulgence in junk food could be a treat for both of you: Make it a special treat! And then turn it into a *slide* or planned *slip* (as we learned in chapter 12), so that you can practice your skills at resisting those cravings.

2. Don't congregate in the kitchen (alteration and avoidance).

Sometime during the 1980's, kitchens became all the rage in the home design world. Island kitchens, eat-in kitchens, restaurant-sized refrigerators, and bar stools at high counters were popping up in everyone's home. But being in the kitchen is a cue for eating, whether you're hungry or not. If you see it, you're more likely to eat it.

Making a habit of congregating in the kitchen is dangerous business. Too many people open their mail in the kitchen, do their homework in the kitchen, talk on the telephone in the kitchen, and on and on. Some people have even put their computer laptop station in their kitchen! And what's going on while they're opening mail, doing homework, talking on the phone, and reading those e-mails? Eating! Eating! Eating!

Instead, stay out of the kitchen as much as you can. It's dangerous in there!

3. Decommission the warehouse-sized pantry (avoidance).

After the fashionable kitchen phase of the 1980's came the monster-pantry-closet phase of the 1990's. With the surge in big box bulk stores came the need for homes with pantries big enough to hold 15-pound boxes of cookies, packages with 75 rolls of toilet paper, and three-gallon squeeze bottles of ketchup. Madness!

People rationalize that they save money by purchasing food in this quantity. That may be true, but for *you* if it's in the house you're much more likely to eat it! If you take that three-pound jar of honey roasted cashews to the couch and pop on the television, do you really need me to tell you what's going to happen next?

Instead, use that closet for something else and resist the urge to buy food in such large quantities. Keep the 75-pack of toilet paper, but get rid of those 15-pound boxes of cookies.

4. Turn off the food cable network (avoidance).

By this point, you probably think I'm a no-fun, militant ogre. Unfortunately, like most of you, I actually love watching all the foodie shows. However, I'm also a realist. And if you're a realist too, it's obvious that watching people cook, prepare and eat food on television is probably not conducive to keeping a nice figure. The commercials on television aren't helping, either. If seeing a 30-second advertisement for nacho chips has been found time and time again to get people off their butts to eat nacho chips, imagine what watching hour upon hour of food television must do!

Instead, find activities aside from watching television to keep you busy. If you must watch television, try to watch programs where food is not the central plot or theme of the show. Watch the exercise channels, home improvement programs, or sports networks instead!

B. Before You Take That First Bite

1. When you're upset and tempted to eat, address what is upsetting you (alteration).

This may be the single most important change you need to make. As you know from chapter 8, *emotional eating* is a huge challenge. I cannot say enough that you must learn methods to deal with emotional upset that don't involve food. There is no food on this earth that genuinely fixes whatever you are upset about, not even chocolate. You know that eating might make you feel a little better for the first two minutes, but it's often followed by feeling much worse for the next 20. Plus, the problem that caused your upset in the first place is still there.

Instead, it would be far better for both your mind and your waistline to sit down with a pad and pencil to work out your feelings, rather than with a bag of cheesy puffs. Read over what you've written and share it with a friend or therapist. Work out what's pushing the eat button. Go back and review the strategies to combat emotional eating in chapter 8.

2. Eating doesn't cure boredom (avoidance).

When we're bored, and can find nothing better to do, we sometimes eat. In fact, this is probably part of the mindless eating autopilot scenario described in chapter 8. When bored, some people's brains just steer them into the kitchen. And while they're deciding what to do, they throw down 275 calories of whatever happens to be lying on the counter.

This would be a good time to change that pattern of behavior. Designate a specific chair or place in your home as your thinking place. Call it your "where-I-go-when-I'm-bored-and-need-to-figure-out-what-I-want-to-do" place. And make sure it's not in the kitchen!

Start to develop new things to do when bored. Buy crossword or other puzzles, play a video game, go for a walk, anything! You would be well served to take eating off of your list of things to do, except for the times when refueling is necessary.

3. Stop cooking for 17 people (alteration).

In my wife's mind, there is no greater crime than inviting people over and not having enough food. To combat this fear, she generally buys enough food just in case the New York Giants show up! Preparing less food at meals is actually a great way to recoup some of the money you're losing by no longer buying the mega-sized cookie package at the big box store.

Instead, consider how many people will be dining and make enough food just for them. If you must, make one extra portion just in case someone brings a friend. This can create a great deal of anxiety in some people. But ask yourself: When was the last time you left your own dinner table and there wasn't enough food? Has this ever happened? If by chance you accidentally made too little, you can always make more. No big deal.

Of course in some cultures, limiting the amount of food on the table would be nothing short of heresy. Being mindful of such cultural traditions while keeping things healthy is certainly possible. When you might not feel comfortable limiting the *amount* of food, you can certainly choose to serve *healthier* food. Grill more vegetables. Serve more salad. Everyone will be happy.

4. Don't serve family style (alteration).

I know that this is sacrilegious for some people because they either grew up with family style serving, they see it as less pretentious and more economical, or they're just too lazy to create individual plate settings. But remember: We see food—we eat food. Seeing and smelling ten portions of delicious food on a huge serving plate that sits only six inches away is just inviting you to eating more.

Instead, prepare a plate in advance for every diner at your table.

By having a preset plate of food, you're more likely to stick to what's in front of you. If other diners want more, invite them to get up and head to the kitchen to refill their platters.

Also, serve on smaller plates. Research shows that using smaller plates results in smaller portions, and people will actually eat less food than when provided with larger plates.

C. Learning New Ways to Eat

1. If you're not hungry, don't eat (avoidance).

You thought we were now going to talk about eating, but hold on for a moment. The primary function of eating food is to provide your body with fuel. Viewing food as fuel and eating as filling up the tank of your car is a helpful analogy. You put gasoline in your car when the car *needs* gas, not when it *wants* gas. Your car doesn't get in the mood for some gas.

Hunger is your body's way of saying that it needs fuel. By eating less and less often, you will become better able to distinguish *needing* food from *wanting* food. Some refer to this strategy as *listening to your hunger*. Admittedly, this approach may steal some of the fun out of eating, but it is the more appropriate way to think about food and eating. Also, if you truly want to lose weight and keep it off, you cannot eat every time you want something.

2. When you want a little something only eat a little something (avoidance).

Perhaps you're hungry or maybe—heaven forbid—you just want a little something even though you're not really hungry. Start by actually having a little something like a small snack, and then wait. If you have one cookie or one pretzel and then wait ten minutes, oftentimes your craving for more will subside.

If you find that you have a hard time keeping your snacks small, then prepare them in advance. Put together small portions of a snack in sealed plastic bags. This way, when you have that craving for a little something, you would simply consume a small bag of pretzels instead of downing an entire box.

By eating a small snack, you had your little something and the consequence was quite minor. And you gave yourself the opportunity to practice a *slide* (chapter 12). Each time you stop at a little something, you learn that you actually *can* stop! You learn that you can choose to control your behavior and that you don't have to avoid food or eating altogether.

3. Eat only at the table (alteration).

Certainly, you've heard this one before. The idea is to combat *mindlessness*, which we learned about in chapter 8. If you're eating while watching the clock or looking out the window or milling around your house, you're not focusing on eating, and that's dangerous.

By sitting at the table and eating *only* at the table, and by doing that over and over again, you're training your brain that this is your eating place. In this way, you're more likely to focus on what you're doing and feeling rather than being distracted by other activities.

4. When eating, do nothing but eat (alteration).

When you're eating, make it a point to do nothing else. Don't eat while reading the paper or while watching television. Don't review your snail mail or e-mail while you're munching. Eating is a pleasure, so try to actually enjoy it.

When you eat while doing other activities you don't even taste what you're eating! It can also lead to mindless eating. By minimizing distractions while you eat, you can focus on eating and all the sensations that go along with it. Some of those sensations will include hints from your stomach that you're full or satisfied. This is one of the body's natural methods to curb eating. Try to listen for it.

5. Put your fork down between bites (alteration).

Putting your fork down will help you slow down your eating. It will also help you avoid loading up the next forkful before you've even finished chewing the previous one.

What's the hurry? By putting the fork down, you're forcing yourself to slow down and concentrate on chewing and enjoying what's in your mouth. I know that you've heard over and over that chewing your food completely before swallowing is important. We tell our children this all the time. But it's especially important for you to master if you want your weight loss surgery to be a success.

6. *Separate eating from drinking (alteration and avoidance).*

Don't wash food down the drain with a drink. When you do, you lose the opportunity to fully taste and savor your food. You also put yourself at greater risk for eating more food than you originally intended.

Instead, chew each bite many times, and completely and take pleasure in what you're eating. An easy method to avoid drinking while eating is to simply not put a glass on the table in the first place. If there's no glass on the table, there's nothing to drink!

7. *Take small bites (alteration).*

Imagine that you're feeding an infant. You want to eat cautiously and mindfully. Put the tablespoon back in the drawer and use a teaspoon instead. In fact, you may want to consider buying a set of toddler's utensils that are available in the baby aisle of your local supermarket. No joke!

If you have a spoon that can only *hold* six pieces of rice, you can *eat* only six pieces of rice at a time. It may sound a bit bizarre, but many patients have told me that this particular recommendation was extremely helpful in learning both to eat smaller bites and to slow down the pace of eating.

D. Learning New Lifestyle Behaviors

1. Exercise (alteration).

I know that you've only heard this seven million times, so I'll say it once more: exercise. But don't just listen to me. Listen to the thousands of people who belong to the National Weight Control Registry, an organization made up of people who have lost at least 30 pounds and kept it off for one year or longer. Almost all of them (95 percent) exercise three or more times per week.

If you're truly serious about keeping that weight off, this means you need to exercise. Don't get hung up on finding the "right" exercise. Find something you enjoy, and then do it as many times a week as you can. You're more likely to keep doing your exercise if you have fun doing it. Because part of your weight loss will happen when you burn more calories, you need to make exercise a part of your new lifestyle to increase your odds of success.

2. Get active (alteration).

Being active involves more than running on a treadmill or using an elliptical machine. It's about *movement*. When you think back to how movement felt at your top weight, everything was difficult and uncomfortable. You may have dreaded simple tasks like going up the stairs or walking around a shopping mall. Now that you can do these things, you should do them often.

Every burned calorie counts, not just those that melt off in the gym. Take even simple opportunities to be more active. Park the car farther away from the entrance to the mall. Walk to do some of your errands, rather than drive. Take the stairs instead of the elevator. Take more active vacations. Take walks on work breaks at the office and at night rather than sitting around the house. All of these little changes will make weight loss easier and improve your health.

3. Defood your brain (alteration).

Some people are what I call *foodies*. Their lives disproportionately revolve around food. They love to cook, watch cooking shows, read cooking books, shop for food, and do almost everything and anything somehow related to food. Some of them acknowledge that this may have been one of the factors that contributed to their obesity.

Now I won't tell you to completely stop being a foodie. But I will tell you that you need to alter your behavior to introduce balance with new things to occupy your time. It is totally necessary that your brain spend less time on food and more time on things other than the future contents of your stomach. Expand your horizons to other interests. Play cards, take a class, volunteer, bike or hike. These are all activities that generally don't involve food. Find something new that works for you.

4. Get social (alteration).

Increasing your social activity means getting out of the house and interacting more with other people. And not just online—I mean in person, in the flesh. Being alone is a major trigger for eating. Anything that puts others around you makes it less likely that you'll be eating. The specific type of social activity you engage in is less important than trying to select activities that don't revolve around food and don't always involve going out to eat. Join a book club, a bowling league, or a yoga class. Find something you enjoy that involves others.

If you can become more social and more active at the same time, even better! Consider joining an active social club, like a local walking or biking group. After you've lost a little weight and your functioning has improved, consider something more energetic like hiking or biking. Making active friends is a great way to ensure that you'll keep the weight off. Your friends will be engaging in the very behavior that you're trying to incorporate into your daily life.

Getting social is so important to weight loss success that I spend the next four chapters talking about it. Read on to learn more!

Part IV

Dealing With Others

We don't live alone. And as much as people may have been mean to you in the past, you still need to deal with them. This section will help you deal—how to dump the bad ones and nurture the good ones. You'll also learn some straight talk to stop folks from throwing those destructive insults. We'll discuss strategies to enhance both platonic and romantic relationships, including how your old relationships can evolve and how your new ones can thrive.

14

Is Everyone Ready For the New You?

"I can't believe how much weight you've lost!"

"You seem so much happier and more confident."

"Congratulations! You did it!"

"You look fantastic!"

"I knew you could do it."

"I'm so proud of you."

HOPEFULLY, YOU CAN RECALL HEARING accolades like these from your friends and family. Perhaps you're still hearing it. Every day seeing someone you haven't seen for a while is a delight rather than a dreadful experience. With each few pounds lost, your appearance, attitude and other qualities have changed a notable degree, prompting continuing compliments from others. You've lost weight and you're starting to feel different about yourself. In general the changes are positive. But sometimes bumps in the road emerge.

"I've heard that a lot of people regain the weight after a few years."

"It's not like you lost the weight. It was the surgery."

"You think you're hot stuff now that you're thin."

"I liked you better before you lost the weight."

"You're so arrogant."

"You took the easy way out."

What's going on? You went through this complete physical transformation and now that you feel better about yourself, you're getting persecuted! Are you really acting that differently than before? Have you become arrogant? You don't think you've changed, but so many people are responding differently, you can't be sure. Why is this happening?

Weight Loss Affects All Your Relationships

As you've probably figured out by now, your physical, emotional and behavioral changes don't occur in isolation. Be aware that changes in you affect every single person around you. Every relationship is like a puzzle with pieces that "learn" to fit into each other as time goes by. In all relationships, each individual plays a role. Think of a role as an expected set of behaviors performed by an individual. It allows us to predict how people will behave and helps us organize our expectations of the people in our lives. We sometimes think of personality in terms of an expected set of behaviors and we describe people this way. When we say that Debbie is shy, what we mean is that Debbie is usually shy and we would expect that she would act this way in a future interaction. When we say Jack is a loudmouth, we mean that Jack has often been one to say what he thinks, even when nobody wants to hear it, and we would expect him to continue to act this way.

In your marriage, at work, with friends, with acquaintances, you may be astounded at just how much losing weight impacts your relationships by changing others' expectations of your behavior. It may appear to you that the only new thing is your waistline, but so much more has changed: your personality, your behavior, the way you think and the role you're willing to play in all of your relationships. You really have become a very different person and everyone notices it. Actually, you may be the last person to truly recognize just how different you are!

There are subtleties that may be unnoticeable to you, but not others. You're probably become a bit more extroverted, talkative and confident. These are positive changes, and the right person will welcome them. But the wrong person may perceive you negatively. It might even take some time for the most accepting folks to become comfortable and accustomed to the new you. How you are received also depends on the role you are playing. Let's look more closely at two major types of relationships.

Marriage and Intimate Relationships

In a marriage, roles evolve over time. One person pays the bills, the other does the food shopping. One person is more responsible for disciplining the kids while the other one handles issues with the neighbors. One person might be more of the decision maker while the other generally defers. When you lose weight and start feeling better about yourself, it is possible that you may want to change or modify some of these roles. For example, you may feel more confident making decisions, which is generally a positive step. But such a step might be met with resistance from your partner. He or she may feel uncomfortable abdicating some responsibilities, as you yearn for more of them.

These are things that need to be worked out. Expect these kinds of changes to emerge over the months as you lose weight. The effect of significant weight loss on intimate relationships is very important and quite complex, and we'll explore such romantic relationships in greater detail in chapter 15.

Friends, Coworkers, and Groups

Individual friendships can change, as well. Most good friends will champion your success. However, in some situations it will alter the relationship. For example, if you have a close friend who has struggled with her weight alongside you, she may start feeling jealous of your success. She may feel like you no longer understand what it's like to struggle with obesity. She may no longer want to talk to you about her weight and efforts to lose weight. She may not want to go clothes shopping with you anymore. She may suddenly feel more self-conscious and reluctant to go out to lunch with you, now that you eat so much less. These may all seem to be small things. But cumulatively they can become major hurdles if not addressed. Sometimes the relationship just works itself out with time. But other times you'll need to put in the effort to assertively address it with your friend.

Group situations become even more complicated, as we are now dealing with a larger cast of characters and personalities. They include your friends, family, and those you encounter at work. Any time we have three or more people in a room, we have a group situation, which operates quite differently from a one-on-one interaction. First, unlike in a one-on-one, it's pretty rare for everyone in a group to function like equals. At work, there are usually delineated roles that are demarcated through specific titles: president, vice president, manager, and the like. The titles are there to illustrate rank and power.

After your weight loss, your overt role in a group may be the same, but the way you'll be treated and addressed by others could be quite different. Groups of friends often function like a small corporation. The members of your group do not have formal titles, but everyone clearly fills a role and has a generally expected set of behaviors. Let's have a little fun and imagine what it would be like if members within a group actually had formal titles.

Every group of friends has its leader or "president," and co-leaders or "vice presidents." The rest of the members are the "employees." The leader of your group is probably extroverted and always proposes what restaurant or movie you're going to on Friday night, or makes the initial suggestion of what gift to buy for someone's baby shower. Some people view her as bossy or pushy, but she does serve her role as the leader of the group. Also consider that she achieved the role of president because others in the group allowed her to.

A few "vice presidents" make up the two or three other people in the group who either agree with the leader or take it upon themselves to challenge the leader and suggest something different. Although they often agree with the leader's perspective, they are comfortable suggesting something else when they want. Finally, the "employees" enjoy being in the group and generally go along with what the president and vice presidents decide. Some may be pushovers, afraid to really rock the boat by suggesting something else, while others simply value the camaraderie of the group and are flexible enough that they don't feel the need to challenge what the majority wants to do. The group continues to exist and function smoothly because the system works, and everybody knows their role and plays it out.

But what happens when someone tries to change her own role? What happens when an "employee" loses 100 pounds and feels more confident and starts acting a bit like a "vice president?" What happens if people *outside* the group start to interact differently with a much thinner and more self-confident person within the group? Things can get sticky in a hurry.

Hopefully, the new you is more confident and comfortable voicing your opinions, and most of your friends allow your role within the group to evolve. However, this change in you has resulted in changes in the way the group operates, as well. Even if the "president" and "vice presidents" of your social group start acting as your cheerleaders, they may be less eager to change their own roles within your group. If they are accustomed to getting much of the attention, either for their opinion or their appearance, at the very least it may feel awkward for them to experience this change in the dynamics of the group. At worst, your friends might be jealous to become show stealers and saboteurs. They might make snide comments or roll their eyes every time someone says how fantastic you look. What do you do?

Common Responses

There are a few different types of responses that people will have towards you regarding your weight loss and the changes in your attitude and behavior. The majority of your friends and family will champion you and celebrate your success. Some may play it cool and make little of your changes, while others may seem to be out-right hostile or jealous of your success. Let's look more closely at the different types of responses you're likely to encounter:

The cheering section.

Hopefully you'll find that most people will have nothing but posi-tive things to say about what you have accomplished. Most of my patients that have lost a great deal of weight enjoy the compliments and increased attention. They are justifiably proud of what they've achieved and most of their loved ones want to let them know that they are, as well.

There are some folks who don't enjoy the increased attention. Others don't mind the attention, but find it anxiety provoking. Some obese people have strong feelings of shame and embarrassment about their size, and when their weight starts to decline and the at-tention increases after surgery, their social skills need some time to catch up. Shy people generally make it a point to avoid the spotlight, so when the spotlight finds them it takes a while to adjust.

Another way to put it is that *fat body* goes away faster than *fat brain*. What this means is that your weight will change much faster than all the other behaviors you are working to change, and in some ways you'll still perceive yourself as weighing much more than you actually do. Fortunately, like most things, practice and repetition will help you become more comfortable with all those new accolades. Eventually, you will actually grow (or is it shrink?) into your new size.

The indifferent.

These folks are not cheering loudly and some may not be cheer-ing at all. That's okay, too! Not everyone is a cheerleader, and believe it or not you may actually enjoy having a few people in your world that don't scream "Oh, my God!" every time you walk into a room. If you've just had surgery, perhaps you'll want the pounds to melt off and for everyone to notice. But I can guarantee that in a few weeks you'll appreciate those folks who are subtler in their acknowledg-ment of your success. While there may be reasons why some don't cheer for you, as long as they don't steal your thunder, it's probably better not to inquire about their reasons for seeming indifferent.

Also, be aware that cheerleaders may become indifferent to your transformation over time, simply because the novelty wears off. A year or so after your surgery, especially if your weight has reached a plateau, the "new you" is just "you." You are no longer "Samantha who lost 85 pounds," you're just "Samantha." This is a good thing. If you're like most people, you had surgery to lose weight and make some changes. And you wanted to keep the weight off so that you could get on with your life. Your goal was either to more fully enjoy the life you had, or to pursue a variety of goals that had been put on the shelf. Now that you're thinner and keeping it off, people are getting used to the new you. There was a time before surgery when you felt out of place, feeling *too* visible or *in*visible. As you lost weight, people eventually got used to the thinner you. It's not that they're no longer impressed or supportive. Rather, the thinner you is now old news.

It's kind of like that brand new red sports car that feels fast, exciting and beautiful. It's got that wonderful new car smell, it's squeaky clean and shiny, and everyone stares as you drive by. You feel like you belong on the cover of the hottest magazine! But in a year's time, that hot sports car is just another car on the road, and you're already looking at the newer models.

This is not necessarily a bad thing. Now you can get on with the business of being the new and improved you with fewer distractions. Hopefully, you didn't lose weight just to have others cheer for you. It was to feel better, look better and to be able to do the things that were difficult so many pounds ago. At this point, you actually may be closer to the end of your weight loss journey than the beginning. Put that car in gear and get on that wonderful road known as weight loss success.

The show stealer.

These are the people in your world who seem to be uncomfortable with what you've accomplished, and they've gone a step beyond indifference. They're violating that familiar social rule that says if you don't have anything nice to say, don't say anything at all. When people start to compliment you, the show stealer rolls her eyes and sighs. When others gather around you to hear your story, the show stealer throws in a subtle (or not so subtle) dig. When you're at a gathering and everyone is commenting on how wonderful you look, the show stealer asserts that you took the easy road or that you somehow cheated.

The show stealer seems uncomfortable with your success and might even do things to sabotage or diminish what you've accomplished, in some ways setting up actual roadblocks in your journey. For example, she's the one always offering you food or trying to encourage you to go off of your eating regimen by having some ice cream with her. Why would a supposed "friend" try to block your progress and what can you do about it?

Let's examine what may be going on here. First, don't assume that these negative comments are completely false or that their accusations are necessarily evil. Consider the fact that you most certainly *have* changed since your dramatic weight loss. Before surgery, you may have been a bit more quiet and reserved. You might not have wanted to draw much attention to yourself. You may have been less confident and outgoing. Now you feel better, look better and have some more confidence. Even if you were an outgoing, bubbly person before surgery, your weight was probably one of the few topics that you shied away from.

After surgery, it's likely that many people are asking you questions about your weight loss, how you did it, and so on. You find yourself in situations where you draw a crowd. Everyone wants to know your secret. Losing as much weight as you have is no small achievement and people want to hear your story. So it's darn likely that you *have* become more talkative, especially about your weight loss surgery story. It's likely that you *are* proud of yourself and you should be. It's quite the achievement! How you speak about your success and tell your story is a critical factor.

Our culture is very interesting when it comes to fame and celebrity. The pattern is predictable. The media initially hypes famous folks, and then delights in demolishing them with dirt just as they reach their peak. They create an image of celebrities as being superhuman and impervious to it all, which of course they never were. And once they show signs of being human with normal foibles, the media sharks devour them. Sadly, we seem all too eager to jump in. Pick any celebrity that you like and you'll see this phenomenon in action: Martha Stewart, Paris Hilton—the list is long.

Why do they want to steal your thunder? I'm going to make a prediction, and it's that most of these folks are either struggling to lose weight themselves, or simply have a high need for the spotlight. You know these folks. They are the queens of gab who always steer the conversation towards themselves. No matter what the conversation, somehow it winds up being about them.

So here you are, at the top of your game, basking in the glory of your success. You've lost the weight, you're wearing the clothes, and hearing how great you look. A word of advice: Be humble. This is not a suggestion that you diminish what you have achieved. Rather, shine a beacon of hope for others, not just a spotlight on yourself. This advice may not prevent the show stealers and saboteurs from coming after you with guns a' blazing, but it will deflect some of the shots.

You can see that we have two types of friends: Those who are still struggling with their weight, and those who need to constantly bask in the glow of attention. Before we deal with each, a caveat: Much of the time these types of interpersonal challenges go away on their own. As people adapt to the changes in you, they acclimate to the changes in the balance of power in your relationships. You are a work in progress, and so are many of your relationships. Even before you lost weight, your relationships were evolving and going through changes here and there. Allow a little time for people to get used to you. In other words, say very little and let it pass. However, if the comments persist or if they escalate, you owe it to yourself to take action with these people. Let's find out how.

Confronting the friend struggling with weight.
It is quite conceivable that this person is more friend than foe. She was likely your partner in crime. This was the friend with whom you commiserated over the months or years about your mutual struggles with weight. Only now, the characters have changed. You are no longer a struggler; you are a victor! Your friend is still fighting the fight and probably feels a bit lonely and betrayed. It's understand-

able: You're standing on the victory mountain while she's left behind fighting the battle. It would not be uncommon to find a bit of insecurity at play. This person feels like a failure and can't see your success as doing anything other than highlighting her own inadequacy. Can you think of a few friends who fit this description?

Your friend sees only two choices: Champion your success or tear you down. By championing your success, she needs to acknowledge that she is still unsuccessfully battling the bulge while you figured it out. By tearing you down, she can maintain the belief that she isn't failing, but rather that you somehow cheated. Or she can tell herself that you won't remain a winner for long. If she jabs at you with snide comments, she can make herself feel better by knocking you down a peg. If you regain the weight, then she is vindicated. If she can attribute your success to surgery rather than effort, she can tell herself that you "cheated" and didn't do it on your own. Of course, this is all nonsense.

One of the most common comments that jealous friends volley across the table is: Well, I'm not ready to take the easy way out. I want to really lose the weight myself. Another common tactic is for her to tell stories about people who have had surgery and gained some or all of the weight back. In either case, these kinds of comments are primarily designed to make her feel better about herself in her own struggle with weight, and not really to attack you.

Although losing weight is not a zero-sum game (as there is no limit to how much total weight loss the world can achieve), it may seem to your friend that if you are a winner, she must be a loser. Naturally, this simply isn't true, but it's easy to see why she might think this way. In fact, there's a good chance that you had these same thoughts in the past when other friends lost weight while you struggled. Human beings seem to have this ridiculous tendency to see everything in such absolute terms: black–and–white, winners and losers, success or failure. Maybe this forced dichotomy makes it easier for us to make sense of the world by sorting everything neatly into two broad categories. Unfortunately, 99 percent of experiences in life are gray, not black nor white.

What to do? You're winning the war and you want your friend to be a winner, as well. Remember to be her beacon of hope. When an overweight friend makes comments that seem to have the intent of cutting you down, what may be happening is that she is indirectly voicing her own struggle with losing weight. Express your understanding of her struggle and make it clear that you are willing to help. As you share your willingness to be there for your friend, you also need to inform her how those negative comments are affecting your relationship with her, and that you want them to stop.

Begin by acknowledging the negative comment, and letting her know that you understand how difficult weight loss can be. You can remind her that you were there with her in the past, and you will remain there in the future. You both went through the diets, the programs, the late night television miracles. Offer to tell her about your story and why you decided to have weight loss surgery. Offer to show her the materials you read to help you make the decision. Let her know that you are willing to answer questions about surgery. This is not to say that you should push or advocate that she should have surgery. Rather, let her know that you completely understand how much of a struggle losing weight can be, and how you decided to address the problem for yourself. Here's how you might say it:

> Janet, I know what you're going through. Do you remember how I did a lot of those diets with you? In fact, we went to some of those meetings together. The small portions, the bags of carrots, I remember it all. But I finally found something that works for me and I've never been happier. I'd really like you to be happy for me, too. Our friendship is so important to me, and I want to help you however I can. But these comments you're making are hurting my feelings. If you're interested in hearing how I made my decision, I'd love to tell you about it. Just let me know when you're ready.

Notice how the person tried to identify with Janet's struggle, reminding her that she's been there, too. She explained her decision and asked for Janet's support. She made herself available to help Janet in her weight loss journey, while also respectfully asking Janet to stop hurting her. You may find it helpful to write down the names (or initials) of those friends who are like Janet, and write some practice conversations. You can work out the conversation in writing first, and later practice it a few times in front of a mirror to make sure you're accurately making your points. This is better than just blurting it out the next time you meet.

Should you try this method of extending an olive branch and find that it's not immediately effective, don't be surprised. The decision to have weight loss surgery is a big one, and most people don't go from hearing about it right to the operating table in a few days. Most give it months of thought before moving forward. In the long run, this is an effective strategy because hundreds of patients have told me that this exact scenario is how they learned about weight loss surgery. And it was this scenario that prompted them to move forward to have the surgery.

Sometimes the negative comments persist, even after the heart-to-heart talk. If so, you owe it to yourself to let your friend know that the comments are inappropriate and hurtful. By saying it in this way, you're informing her that her behavior is damaging the friendship. If she's truly friend, it should bother her to learn that she's hurting you, and this might motivate her to change.

If your friend does not respond to your offers of help, and the negative comments show no signs of subsiding, you must reconsider whether she is truly a friend. Friends don't make it a habit to make repeated snide comments that hurt those they profess to love. Given all that you've gone through, you owe it to yourself to surround yourself with people who want what is best for you and have your best interests in mind. Sometimes you have to cut ties with people who no longer meet these requirements.

Before you take such drastic action, be sure to give it some time. Many times these friends will come to recognize their jealousy and their inappropriateness towards you and apologize.

Confronting the spotlight hog.

The spotlight hog is probably not one to help, and may be the one to ignore. The spotlight hog has their own insecurities, and almost like a plant needs the constant glow of the light for her fragile ego to survive. With such folks, you are not necessarily a threat because of your thinness. Rather, you are a threat because your success takes them out of the limelight.

For the spotlight hog, the topic of conversation is almost always themselves. They talk for the sake of talking, which is usually fine, unless they're also trashing you. Generally, these folks are more bark than bite. They are a refined version of the playground bully, but they do it with Gucci and Prada and references to whom they know and where they've been rather than fists and sticks.

How should you approach the spotlight hog? Your best move in the short run may be to say and do nothing. Give them a chance to learn that you're not stealing the limelight, merely borrowing it for a while. Once she determines that you're not a threat, she'll probably turn her attention elsewhere. If the spotlight hog happens also to be overweight, try the strategies we discussed earlier in this chapter.

After you've given this person several opportunities to get over your success, and after you've tried to ignore her comments over and over, you may find that your efforts have failed. If so, you'll need to speak up. Keep in mind that she's like a playground bully. And like most adult bullies, she is best quieted through polite, private confrontation. What's important for her to understand is that you're not going to sit idly by and take it. This usually works. Consider this approach:

> Marcie, I've sat here for months listening to your rude comments about me, and I've politely asked you several times to stop. I'm now insisting that they stop. Your comments are rude and hurtful and I can't understand why you, a friend, would say such horrible things to me. I want you to really give some thought to how you've been behaving toward me and why you've been acting this way ever since I lost my weight. I want you to know that I would really like to keep you as a friend and work this out. If you want to talk about it more, I'm ready to listen. But I'm not simply going to ignore it any longer.

In this way, you're confronting your friend by putting her on notice. You've let Marcie know what the problem is and what you want her to do about it. You're making yourself available for further discussion, but have made it clear that her behavior is not negotiable: You're not going to take it any more. Like with the earlier scenario of Janet, you may find it helpful to identify your own friends who are like Marcie, and then write and rehearse some practice conversations.

You may wonder whether you should even bother keeping a person like Marcie in your life. It's important to understand that you should not rush to judgment. Remember that you have changed, and it will take some time for others to get used to the new you. And remember that there might be a chance for you to be a beacon of hope to your friend, to help her with her own weight loss struggles.

Going Forward With the New You

Unfortunately, there may be relationships that truly cannot be fixed. Such relationships may always have broken parts. No matter how often you try to fix things, it doesn't work out. All your constructive efforts to get certain friends to stop the negative comments seem to fail. Things you used to be able to talk about with them are now taboo. You may decide to keep such people around, but their role in your life will certainly be diminished, or at least become different. You'll need to think of it as their loss.

Make a promise to yourself that you will not compromise your self-esteem simply to keep certain people in your life. *Do not compromise on becoming the person you wish to become.* Do not allow other's negativity and insecurity to interfere with your positive changes and ongoing personal development. However polite you wish to be, make it clear through your statements and your actions that the folks who wish to remain in your life essentially have no choice but to accept the new you. The old you is gone.

Remember some of those things you wanted to accomplish by losing weight? The opportunity to pursue new relationships with more confidence and comfort was probably somewhere on your list. Now is the time to bring new people into your life, people who have the potential to enhance and improve your life. It is often said that we can't pick our family, but we can certainly choose our friends. Choose wisely!

Rest assured that over time, all of your relationships will sort themselves out. Relationships are always works in progress, and after surgery you may be going through a period of rapid and unexpected relationship changes. Make ongoing efforts to discuss these changes with your friends and family. This is how they thrive. This is how you thrive. By making yourself available to discuss these issues, you will not only be making positive changes in yourself, but in your loved ones, as well.

15

Dating, Intimacy, and Romantic Relationships

RAMATIC WEIGHT LOSS CAN HAVE a significant effect on intimate relationships. For many, the weight lost through surgery allows people who have avoided intimate relationships to begin pursuing one. For others, the weight lost through surgery provides the impetus to make changes in their existing intimate lives. Without question, changes in intimate relationships is one of the more common issues discussed on weight loss surgery Internet chat rooms. It is certainly one of the most common topics discussed in my chat room—my office, that is!

Prior to having surgery, many patients admit that their desire for an intimate relationship is a major motivation for considering weight loss surgery. A number of patients have indicated that they have completely avoided such relationships because of shame and embarrassment regarding their body. Others have said that they would never want to be in a relationship with someone who would want them at their current weight. In my professional view, the lack of an intimate relationship or the lack of intimacy in an existing relationship is one of the most common and damaging effects that obesity has on the quality of life among my patients.

Some folks are in an unsatisfying intimate relationship, and are looking forward to losing the weight to make changes in these relationships. Sometimes the changes are desirable and expected, such as when one partner in a relationship starts to feel better about her body and is more receptive to physical intimacy. Other times the changes are unexpected or potentially damaging, such as when one partner in a relationship starts to feel better about himself and begins to engage in extramarital relationships, or when one partner in a marriage begins to contemplate dissolving the marriage now that she feels that "she can do better."

A few patients have disclosed that they married their spouse primarily because their partners expressed an interest in them as opposed to their own genuine love and affection for their partners. When the weight came off, they now wanted to go out and find if "they can do better." While this is not necessarily a poor decision, it is certainly one that requires a great deal of thought and reflection. Done impulsively, ending relationships is often quite destructive.

What Is an Intimate Relationship?

By *intimate relationship*, I am referring to a loving, partnered romantic relationship. Such a relationship is one that likely includes both emotional and physical components. Intimate relationships are often sexual relationships, but not always. If you are a man, you can now understand why your wife becomes frustrated with you every time she says she wants more intimacy in the relationship and your first impulse is to lunge at her from across the bed.

Many of my patients blushingly admit that they were reluctant to tell me that their interest in pursuing an intimate relationship was one of the major reasons they wanted surgery, believing it to be an inappropriate reason to have the surgery. Why? What's wrong with wanting to be in a loving relationship? How is that somehow a bad thing? Isn't it a pity that people have been made to feel ashamed of their desire to be in an intimate relationship?

Reality Check

Intimate relationships are one of the true joys of life and being morbidly obese makes finding a mate much more difficult. Yes, it is true that people *should* be more focused on "inner beauty," but your appearance is the first impression you make on other people, and it seems that most folks find morbid obesity to be less attractive than having an appropriate body weight.

I was over 210 pounds in high school. The girls were not lining up outside my door. However, the jocks and the really good-looking guys had no trouble finding a date for the prom. It seems that whatever my positive qualities were, they weren't doing much in the way of attracting the opposite sex.

Human beings are social creatures. Ever notice how most of us elect to live in cities or suburbs with lots of people around? Most folks try to make friends with others and enjoy spending time with them. And most pursue intimate relationships with others. It's normal. It's natural. It's healthy. It's truly unfortunate that a morbidly obese person would feel ashamed to admit that they desire an intimate relationship, something that's completely normal and natural.

Obesity affects sexual performance, and might very well affect desire and libido, as well. So there's no need for shame or embarrassment when acknowledging that you're hoping that dropping the weight adds some oomph to your sex life. When a patient tells me part of the reason they want to have surgery is to help them pursue an intimate relationship, I view her as a person who is ready to move ahead with her life. I'm thrilled that she's ready get off the sidelines and into "the game." But I also know that for many, "the game" can be quite terrifying.

Obesity and the Single Girl

The majority of patients who express concerns about intimate relationships are female. This may be because men are more reluctant to discuss these concerns than women. However, the real issue is likely that it's harder to be obese, single and female than it is to be obese, single and male. For better or worse, in our society it's easier being the "big guy" than the "big girl." You may meet a guy who is championed for his ability to eat 15 hot dogs in ten minutes. I strongly doubt any woman will tout her prowess in this area. Men have beer bellies or a paunch, which many people seem to accept. However, women are not given such cute labels, and it's hard to find any wiggle room for females when it comes to a few extra pounds.

Many of the obese women I have seen report that they haven't been in an intimate relationship for many years, or have had the occasional date, though nothing serious. The most common concerns expressed are fears of rejection and humiliation. Hundreds of patients have shared painful stories of their dating attempts, where after first sight the possibility of intimacy is quickly extinguished. Here's what I hear on a daily basis:

> "I haven't even *thought* about dating for years."

> "I've had a hundred first dates, but no second dates. I don't think I can take that again."

> "I wouldn't want to be with anyone who would want to be with me."

> "I can't stand myself this way. I can't imagine how someone else could."

> "Are you kidding me? With this body?"

Obesity Within a Romantic Relationship

There are also many folks I see who are in an intimate relationship, but feel that true intimacy and the connection with their partner has been absent for many years.

> "I make my husband leave the room when I get undressed."

> "We stopped having sex *years* ago. Then we stopped touching. And now it's as if we are just roommates."

> "We've become an old married couple. But we're not old and I barely feel married."

> "I still love her. But the spark isn't what it once was."

> "My snoring got so bad that I now sleep in the den."

Clearly, these comments are not exclusive to those battling morbid obesity. Sadly, I hear them almost every day. It's pretty obvious that weight has a profound impact on the quality of intimate relationships. So it's only natural that so many people look forward to losing weight to address these problems. However, as much as weight loss is sought after, many are nervous about the changes that may occur following such dramatic weight loss. Not everyone is in the same type of intimate relationship and not everyone has the same expectations or hopes regarding the changes that will ensue following weight loss surgery.

Types of Relationships

It's hard to prescribe a one size fits all set of guidelines to address intimate relationships that evolve as a result of weight loss surgery. There are as many relationships as there are couples, and the unique circumstances of each individual always need to be taken into account. Nonetheless, to help us make some sense of the infinite possibilities, it's possible to identify a few types of pre-surgical relationship situations commonly seen:

1. You are not in an intimate relationship, but really want to be.

2. You are in a relationship, but feel it's not very satisfying.

3. You are in a relationship, and feel that you are satisfied.

4. You are not particularly interested in pursuing an intimate relationship.

You probably fit into one of these scenarios prior to embarking on weight loss surgery. Let's look at each in a bit more detail.

You Aren't In an Intimate Relationship, But Really Want To Be

Without question, the majority of single patients that I meet fall into this category. Most report that they haven't made much effort in recent years because they're uncomfortable with their appearance. But they're eager to start after they lose some weight.

Self-esteem is clearly suffering here. If you were ever in this scenario, you would probably agree. Thankfully, losing weight generally provides a tremendous boost to self-esteem, and often allows you to gradually venture back into the waters of dating and intimacy. This is the time when you can rely on friends who are eager to set you up on a date with folks they know. Or you can take advantage of online resources, singles events, or parties to meet people. The process often moves slowly, so don't be discouraged if it takes time. But if you're serious and purposeful about entering a new romantic relationship, chances are good that you'll wander into Mr. or Ms. Right.

Overcoming dating anxiety.

Some folks are rather surprised to find that they're a bit more anxious with dating than they expected. Such anxiety is quite normal and consistent with the fact that this is a new and exciting experience. If you haven't been in the dating world for some time (or ever), it's perfectly understandable to have some anxiety. What do I say on the first date? Will I know what to do if things progress? What will he think of my body? These are common and understandable questions that generate a moderate level of trepidation. You might need little more than the usual encouragement and support of friends and family, so seek it out. Keep in mind that this is the opportunity that you've been waiting for!

Some folks haven't dated for so long that their anxiety almost paralyzes them into inaction. They are very anxious about the entire business of dating and admit that dating is their biggest fear. This fear can stem from a number of sources. Some feel poorly equipped to start meeting new people. Others have friends who are eager to push them out onto the dating scene, but fear they won't be ready. And others simply don't know how to behave on a date because they're rusty and so out of practice.

A few folks just cannot overcome anxiety regarding intimate relationships as they lose weight, sometimes related to past histories of physical or sexual abuse. If this is the case, professional help is clearly warranted. There is no shame in seeking professional help to assist with the anxiety of dating.

On the bright side, it's been my experience that most people find losing a great deal of weight does seem to make things easier for them. This will probably be the case for you, as well. You will no longer be as terrified, and your anxiety will be more manageable than you originally feared. Sooner or later, you've got to go on that date. You will do just fine!

Learning or relearning dating skills.

Dating skills? Are there really such things as dating skills? You bet! You may not realize it, but dating is definitely a skill. When you were in high school, you were thrown to the wolves. You learned dating skills by trial and error. Some people were good at dating and others were not. If you've never really dated or it's been years since you've been out there, you might need to freshen up some of those dating skills in order to feel comfortable again. You may also need to learn a few new ones.

In today's world, it's quite common for people to have coaches for interviewing, and there are thousands of articles written every year on interviewing skills and tactics. Well, if you think about it, a first date is simply an interview for a relationship. If you do well on successive interviews (dates) you wind up getting accepted for the position of partner in the relationship!

Just as there are interview coaches in the professional world to help you find jobs, there are dating coaches, image consultants, and a gamut of other professionals who can help you improve your dating skills. It may sound strange that a successful person who's running a corporation would be baffled by something as simple as dating, but it's not unusual. Making decisions about running a business is quite different from making decisions about intimate relationships. In business, there is generally far less emotion on the line. Many folks share that the business decisions are much easier for them because, after all, it's only money!

Another difference between work decisions and dating decisions is that the successful businessperson's skills are well rehearsed over a number of years across a variety of situations. However, their dating skills may never have been developed or practiced, and can be quite rusty. Many folks can't recall where to go or what to talk about on a date. Do we meet for coffee or dinner? Do I pay or do I let him pay? Others tell me that they're not sure what to do if the date goes well. Do I take him back to my place or should I hold back? Do I allow a good night kiss or not on the first date? Some have been overweight since childhood, and have never dated. It can all be quite overwhelming.

For most people, dating skills develop in adolescence and evolve naturally. However just like any other skill, if they aren't practiced they are quickly diminished. Take flirting, for example. The hair tossing, the coy glances, the batting of eyelashes, the body posture. Maybe you remember flirting as a younger person or have seen others flirting. None of this behavior is random. It may be somewhat hard wired, but it's clearly enhanced by learning experiences. Perhaps you've never thought of it this way, but what humans do in a singles bar is absolutely no different than what you see peacocks, insects, bears, and dolphins doing on the television nature channels. These are behaviors designed to attract a mate. If you're not good at them, you don't get a mate. So it's important to make the development and practice of dating skills a priority.

There are many types of dating skills, including how to dress, how to talk, what to say, and what not to say. Many people hate playing games when dating. But that's exactly what dating is: a game. I don't mean this disparagingly, of course. And I'm not trying to belittle or make fun of courtship. However dating is fun (like a game), it requires certain skills (like a game), and you get better with practice (like a game). In fact, if viewed in the context of the nature channels, it's more like a competitive sport than a game! A singles event is no different than a football game with players, equipment, a field, you name it. So it's important to learn and practice some of these skills as you move forward with dating.

A common question about dating is, "Where can I meet people?" In years past, many met their partner in school or work. Why? Because these are the two places where most people spend the majority of their time. No additional effort is involved in finding a place. You're there; they're there, so it's perfect! These are great places to start looking. But if these two places don't work out, you need to expand your dating arena. This is true whether you're attempting to meet Mr. Right or simply trying to make new friends. If there's nobody in your office that suits your taste, then you need to make an effort to find and go to other places to meet new people.

While I'm encouraging you to develop some of these skills, you don't really do it by venturing back to high school. You do it today by going on dates. Recognize that while you may not have dated in a while, you probably do have friends. And many of the social skills you use with friends overlap with those you would use on a date. This means that most of what you *need* to know, you already *do* know.

Whatever gaps exist in your dating skills, and whatever skills are rusty, will best be acquired and oiled by venturing out there with the love and support of friends and family. Should you need a little extra assistance, remember that there are thousands of dating support groups out there. And there's always the option of professional help, if necessary.

You Are In a Relationship, But Feel It's Not Very Satisfying

Folks in this group appear to be the most anxious because they feel that something needs to change. They want to shake up the status quo, and this involves changes in the behavior of their partner who may not be so interested in changing. If it turns out that your partner is eager to improve the relationship, great progress can be made. The two of you can either give it a shot without outside help, or you could try some intervention such as couples, marital or sex therapy. However, if your partner is not so interested in changing, the work can be far more difficult. We'll talk more about that possibility later.

Occasionally a patient confides that she's in an unsatisfying intimate relationship, and wonders whether she'll become increasingly dissatisfied with the relationship after surgery. Her questions demonstrate that losing weight might upset the apple cart, acknowledging that losing weight could be the easier part of weight loss surgery. I've met several patients in emotionally unsatisfying or abusive relationships who stay put simply because they don't believe they could find a better partner, even at their new lower weight. While I will passionately dispute their doubts, few have any intention of leaving their relationship, and even fewer express much hope in finding a better one.

After surgery, the balance of power in a bad relationship may begin to change. The now thinner partner feels better about herself and becomes more assertive, changing the dynamic within the relationship. She no longer settles for business as usual. Such role changes are very similar to what we see happening in friendships (chapter 14), where an "employee" in a friendship group might begin behaving more like a "vice president."

If the patient's partner is receptive and not threatened by this change, it can take the relationship to a higher level and allow for a greater connection and much deeper intimacy. Relationships often become renewed. Many patients confided that their improved self-esteem and body image reignited their relationship and made it seem more like it was when the couple first met. This, of course, is the "happily ever after" ending to the weight loss journey.

But sometimes the reverse occurs. If the partner is threatened by the now thinner mate's invigorated sense of self and assertiveness, and prefers the former arrangement where they may have been more dominant, conflict can occur. With improved self-esteem, the formerly obese mate may begin to detach and look outside the relationship for both emotional and physical intimacy. Some simply leave the relationship. In the long run this may turn out to be the correct move. However, if changes are made impulsively without forethought, major problems can ensue.

On a few occasions, I've had a patient who impulsively walked out the door. Unless this is an abusive relationship, this is almost always a poor decision because the problems within the relationship may have been reconcilable. At the very least, there is no closure. Sometimes the person leaving doesn't realize that their weight wasn't the only factor in the deterioration of the relationship, and by leaving they're simply taking their problem with them. Under these circumstances, there is a high likelihood that they'll bring those problems into the next relationship. If this occurs, they'll be quite depressed and anxious, believing that leaving their previous partner was a mistake, often a decision that cannot be undone. Even when leaving is the best choice, it should be done with prudence and preparation. There are emotional, legal, financial and other considerations one should take into account before exiting a long-term relationship, especially when children are involved.

It's critical to initiate a peaceful and rationale dialogue with your partner. Have your conversations in a neutral location like at a café.

Make lists about each of your priorities in the relationship, and see if you can come to some agreement. Certainly assert your desires and wishes, but also be willing to compromise. There have likely been a number of changes in you, your partner and in your intimate relationship, and all of your futures are at stake. Both of you are probably aware of this and need to acknowledge what's going on so that careful and productive decisions can be made.

Psychological counseling would certainly be helpful to sort out these complicated and often confusing issues. If the counseling yields no improvement in the relationship, arrangements can then be made to end the relationship under better terms than simply walking out the door. Sometimes couples turn to a mediator to help work through the complex process of terminating a marriage, so that the couple can do so amicably and without thousands of dollars in legal fees spent haggling over petty issues.

You Are In a Relationship, and Feel That You Are Satisfied

If you're part of this group, then after weight loss surgery you will probably find that what is already good just gets better. You're more able to participate in activities with your partner and the world is a bigger and more fulfilling place. You now can do things you only dreamed of before.

But there are challenges. You might find that your partner is struggling to adjust to all of the changes in you. After losing the weight, you might think and feel that you're exactly the same person with a smaller body, but that's not the case. Plus the changes in you have likely created changes in your partner, as well. While this is all generally a positive outcome, it still involves change that can tax your intimate relationship. Change, for better or worse, is stressful.

Sometimes, these issues just work themselves out. After losing weight, you may be more outgoing, more assertive, or more adventurous. Your partner may just need some time to get used to the changes in you. It's always a good idea to keep the channels of communication open. One way to help your partner get used to the changes in you would be to ask how those changes are affecting him or her. Make it clear that you recognize that changes in you can affect your partner, as well. Ensure that your partner feels comfortable talking to you about it.

You Are Not Particularly Interested In Pursuing an Intimate Relationship

At first glance, you would think these folks would have the least amount of anxiety. They're not in a relationship and say that they like it that way. Nothing needs to change and they can remain in their interpersonal comfort zone, even as they lose the weight. They view the weight loss from surgery as being tremendously liberating, allowing them to pursue their interests outside of the dating realm.

Interestingly, with a little time, these folks are frequently surprised to find that they're more interested in intimate relationships than they thought they would be. Perhaps they pushed the idea to the back of their mind when they were obese to avoid the pain of longing for something they believed impossible. Or perhaps they began to feel lonely, again. Or maybe they addressed the anxieties that made them avoid dating. Regardless, folks who initially see themselves in this group usually don't stay there for very long. Eventually they leave this group, and join others in search of a romantic partner.

The Snow Globe

The intent of this chapter is not give the impression that losing a lot of weight always creates havoc in your intimate relationships. For many solid relationships, it makes a good thing even better. And there are certainly times when partners just roll with the punches, and despite all the changes things work themselves out over time.

I keep a snow globe on my desk—you know, that glass bubble with the lighthouse in it that makes it look like it's snowing when you shake it. The snow globe provides a good analogy for the effects of weight loss surgery on your life. Prior to surgery, all the snow is set in place and your life is relatively predictable, which is true for most people whether they are heavy or thin. After losing weight, the globe gets shaken and things may seem topsy-turvy for a while. Your job is different, eating is different, socializing feels different, and people treat you differently. After a while, the snow begins to resettle and there is a new normal, one that is hopefully better than before. Remember that losing weight creates opportunities for you to make changes. Some of these opportunities happen, whether you wanted them to or not. Therefore, it's advisable to anticipate these possibilities, as well as understand and prepare for them.

Many folks who are in relationships discuss these concerns with their partner when they are first thinking about having surgery. By and large, this is a good idea. Generally, they do so to seek support and approval for the decision to have the surgery. They recognize that although they may be the one having surgery, it's going to impact their partner, as well. A partner that expresses support and encouragement of you before surgery is more likely to be supportive of many of the behavioral and emotional changes you experience after surgery. The journey is a long one, and it's nice having a partner along for the ride.

16

Straight Talk: Becoming More Assertive

THE WORLD DOESN'T LIKE OVERWEIGHT people. There, I've said it. It's not pretty, but it's absolutely true. Discrimination against the obese is widespread. I've been there myself. The demeaning treatment takes its toll. Most people's self-esteem and self-image suffer due to their weight. Many also describe how their weight has impacted their intimate and social relationships, as well as their careers.

Therefore, overweight people have to develop some pretty strong coping strategies to make it through their days without going off the deep end. Some of these strategies are not the best approaches to take, but they're common among folks who battle with their weight. Each strategy has temporary advantages, which is why they exist in the first place. But in the long run, they have significant disadvantages because they erode your self-esteem and self-respect. Three of the most prevalent undesirable strategies involve:

1. Trying to be humorous around others, coming across as the *funny guy*.
2. Tolerating mistreatment from others by being the *doormat*.

3. Being bitter and angry with others, keeping them at a
distance to become the *loner*.

Sometimes these strategies make overweight folks appear as if
they possess a particular personality trait. But ascribing a "personality" to someone can be misleading. A person isn't always the funny
guy, or always the doormat. Some people may have naturally developed an interpersonal approach that is an amalgam of all three
coping strategies. Others may adopt different coping techniques de-
pending on the social circumstances. For example, you may have
learned that being funny never works with your friend Bob. He's just
too domineering and you seem more likely to play the role of doormat when he's around. But with your kid brother, being the funny
guy seems most effective. Over time and repetition you're probably
going in and out of these roles so naturally that you don't even recognize you're doing it.

Learning to Cope

Perhaps the hardest part of becoming more assertive is trying to
overcome these roles, because assertiveness involves *challenging* other
folks' negative perceptions of you. Being the funny guy, the doormat
or the loner are unproductive coping strategies, and they don't challenge the other's negative perceptions. But before you *learn* how to
challenge those perceptions with the new coping technique of assertiveness, you'll need to *unlearn* these old unproductive strategies. And
that's not always easy.

These unproductive coping mechanisms were primarily learned
over time to help you adapt to your social environment. Of course
by "learned" I don't mean you voluntarily went to school to become
a professional comedian. Rather, the learning occurred more gradually over the course of your life. When you tried to be funny, you
found that it temporarily deflected negative attention away from
your weight, and that made you feel better. The behavior of being
humorous became stronger (*reinforced* is the technical term) by your
social environment, and so was more likely to happen in the future.
This is very similar to the concept of Darwin's *natural selection* (from
his book, *On the Origin of Species*) as applied to your individual cir-

cumstances. These coping mechanisms developed so that you could compete socially.

Let's look more closely at how this can happen. How could a fat kid get through his day with the least amount of emotional injury? Think of all of those teenage, high school movies you've watched over the years. In these movies we routinely see fat kids, nerds, geeks, and all of the other social misfits mercilessly picked on by the bullying jocks and the beautiful, popular kids. Those of us who identify with one of the misfits love it when the underdog wins. We love it when the geek gets the prom queen or when the nerd outperforms the jock. Unfortunately, this is not what usually happened in school, which is why it's so gratifying to see it play out on the big screen.

So, how did the fat kid get through the merciless gauntlet of hallways in the high school? He was funny, a doormat or a loner. If you commonly dealt with bullies by being funny when you were a kid, your tendency to use humor became stronger. If bowing your head and walking away without saying a word was how you dealt with difficult people, then being a doormat was reinforced for you. After several years and thousands of repetitions of engaging in such coping mechanisms, and meeting with the short term positive consequences of their use, these behaviors have become second nature. Just like with *mindless eating* (chapter 8), you're now engaged in *mindless coping*—you may not even be aware you are doing it!

The main reason to modify these coping strategies is that you don't like how you are behaving and that you want to change. I'm not suggesting that you altogether abandon these strategies. Do not abandon your great sense of humor, for example. Rather, I'm asking you to become more mindful of your coping behaviors, and to decide whether engaging in those behaviors is really the best way to address your weight. To help you decide, let's look a little more closely at each of these roles.

The Funny Guy

It may seem to be a stereotype, but I can attest to the fact that a lot of overweight people are funny. Whether morbidly obese people are significantly funnier than thin people is uncertain, but I've spent a great number of hours laughing on the job. Unfortunately, the

humor is often self-deprecating. It's a Darwinian adaptive strategy—
survival of the funniest. Obese patients and others describe two
functions that the self-deprecating humor of the *funny guy* can serve:

1. I cut myself down before you have a chance, which pro-
   tects me while at the same time disarming you.
2. Humor endears me to you because people often like the
   funny guy. The strategy is simple: My sense of humor is a
   characteristic you might find attractive should you find my
   appearance to be unattractive.

Heavy people should abandon this strategy, if for no other reason than it generally backfires in the long run. This strategy only
persists because of the reinforced temporary benefit. It's probably
less likely that others will insult you now that you've just insulted
yourself. However the irony is that in the long run it'll probably
make others feel more comfortable insulting you, given that you've
demonstrated that you're seemingly comfortable with it. Even if you
convince yourself that you're okay with these barbs, I would argue
that you shouldn't be. In either case they serve to erode your self-esteem. Some might argue that you eventually get used to it. However,
most patients convey that if they tell (or hear) fat jokes often enough,
they start to believe them. It becomes a *self-fulfilling prophecy*, where
you start to believe things you hear over and over, even though they
aren't true (similar to what we discussed about being powerless or
lazy in chapters 9 and 11).

The Doormat

The *doormat* is basically the funny guy without the sense of humor. He just takes it all in: the jokes, the comments, the sneers, the
constant diet suggestions, and on and on. He says very little and
usually bows his head and walks away. The doormat is afraid of conflict. He's afraid that more belittling is just around the corner. He's
afraid of further embarrassment. He generally has low self-esteem
and may believe that he actually deserves poor treatment from others because he's overweight.

Like the funny guy, the doormat believes many of the comments thrown at him and is often quite depressed. He might be more isolated than the funny guy because he lacks the strategy of humor to win over others. However, the doormat may have a cadre of friends, most of whom are also doormats.

It's very likely that you can trace the beginnings of being a doormat back to adolescence. In every high school there are groups or cliques. The doormats are often an amalgam of nerds, geeks, new kids, fat kids, and other eccentrics. They are from the land of misfit toys, like the classic character Rudolph, from *Rudolph the Red-Nosed Reindeer* by Robert Lewis May. They may feel like outsiders in comparison to the beautiful, popular kids. But within their own group they probably have a strong sense of belonging. Nevertheless, they are likely to experience feelings of loneliness, fear and self-loathing when they are around the "beautiful people." And these feelings are carried with them into adulthood.

The Bitter and Angry Loner

The bitter and angry *loner* doesn't take a lot of garbage from others. He dishes it out! This person is angry at the world and fends others off, not through humor, but by being a bear. The bitter and angry loner doesn't want to be endearing. Rather, he wants to keep others away from him. The strategy goes something like this: I'll hit you before you hit me! While this does defend him from other people's comments and opinions, he's not having a particularly good time of it, and being bitter and angry isn't truly helping his self-esteem.

This type of patient will tell me that other people are mean and nasty and that he's okay being a loner because there's nobody in the world that's worth his time anyway. The problem is that he doesn't really believe this. He desperately wants to be proven wrong and to have meaningful relationships with others. As you might expect, it's not easy for him to make new friends. He doesn't want to get hurt so he is defensive, making it difficult to get close to him.

Unlike the funny guy or the doormat, the bitter and angry loner probably has no misfit group he can call his own. As a kid, he was probably very anxious, isolated and did his own thing. He may very well have had no friends or perhaps just one or two. At some point, unlike the funny guy or the doormat, he probably stopped trying to find his way through social circles and kept to himself. His family may have been his only real social connection, if that. The bitter and angry loner is a most unhappy soul. And of all the coping strategy characterizations, the loner will likely be the most difficult to turn around because his social skills and faith in the good of others are the most compromised.

Fat Body versus Fat Brain

I am known for telling my patients that weight loss surgery will take care of *fat body* long before it does anything for *fat brain*, a concept introduced in chapter 14. Put simply, you'll lose weight much faster than you'll lose the perception that you're overweight, and faster than you'll repair the damage that being overweight has caused. For many patients, being overweight was a major ingredient in the formation of their personality's coping styles, and personality doesn't change so quickly.

Sometimes, these coping styles decline gradually with reductions in weight. But more often it takes hard work for them to change. It's imperative that you engage in this work to accelerate the process. In theory, the task is rather simple: Act as if you were thinner and your fat brain will catch up with your thinner body. Think about how people who are not concerned about their weight act in social situations, and then simply act as if you were one of them. Of course it's not as easy as it sounds. But it doesn't have to be terribly complicated either, so read on for some pointers.

Assertiveness

The coping strategy to replace the funny guy, the doormat or the loner is called assertiveness. There are a number of definitions of *assertive*, and volumes have been written on the subject. Put simply, if you behave assertively it means that you're communicating in such a way as to defend your rights and pursue your goals, while respecting the rights and goals of others. Assertiveness, like all forms of communication, is both verbal and nonverbal; you're communicating by both what you say and what you do. By being assertive, you're demonstrating to others that you think well of yourself and expect others to treat you with the same kind of respect that they would want from you. Being assertive means speaking directly and honestly. Being assertive does not mean that you are cocky or arrogant. In fact, you can be assertive and quite friendly. You're simply displaying self-respect through your words and actions.

Sometimes it's helpful to contrast assertiveness with the two other types of behavior: passivity and aggression. When you're *passive*, it means that you're sacrificing your rights and goals for the benefit of others. But when you're *aggressive*, you're sacrificing others' rights in the pursuit of your own wishes and goals. Put another way, passivity occurs when you allow yourself to get trampled upon by others (like being a doormat) while aggression happens when you're trampling over others in pursuit of your own objectives. Assertiveness is the win-win scenario. That's not to say that everyone is always happy when you're assertive, but the intention is that nobody gets hurt.

You may be wondering where passive-aggressiveness falls into the scheme of things. *Passive-aggressive* is a term that is very commonly used to refer to those who don't say what they want to say directly or promptly, but then are inappropriately sharp at a later point. Those who are passive-aggressive do not have the ability to say or do what needs to be said and done in the moment, so they come back for the kill at a later time. Passive-aggressiveness is cowardly and is therefore really another form of passivity.

Let me give you a good example: When I taught college courses, I invited students to meet with me during office hours to discuss their grades. I also offered students the opportunity to request and complete an extra credit assignment to help boost their grades. One student was unhappy with his grade, but chose not to discuss it with me or to request an extra credit assignment. Instead he vandalized my car, which was discovered when a fellow student told me of his behavior. Notice: He passively said nothing but then aggressively vandalized my car. His actions were cowardly.

Perhaps the most common example of passive-aggressiveness is *sarcasm*. Sarcasm is the official language of passive-aggressiveness. It involves saying something without really saying it directly. It is snide and has the intent to harm or hurt the recipient, without seeming to do so directly. Most people who use sarcasm are afraid to say what needs to be said directly, in a way that would make them accountable and would require them to discuss their opinions. Instead they throw darts. They are frightened bullies. They are passive.

I should note that I've met my share of heavy people who were comfortable being assertive before they had surgery and lost weight. They are the ones who refuse to hide in shame and make excuses to the rest of the world. These folks acknowledge their size but refuse to allow it to be an excuse for mistreatment by others. They simply do not allow an entire social interaction to devolve solely because of their weight. They respect themselves too much to allow that to happen. They view their weight as one aspect of themselves, but not one that justifies shame and abuse from others. After weight loss surgery, these folks adjust rather quickly and often report feeling whole again. Such patients tell me that their image in the eyes of others is apparently now commensurate with their appearance. They act like they deserve respect, and they now look the part.

Getting to Work

Now it's time to learn some constructive coping strategies. The bitter and angry loner has been avoiding people or yelling and aggressively screaming at others to get them to back off. He needs to try and tone things down a bit and learn to play more nicely with others. The funny guy and the doormat have been passively avoiding confrontation by either laughing things off or simply ignoring them. They need to learn to address others more directly and stop letting things slide.

Clothes shopping is a perfect opportunity to practice becoming more assertive. When shopping for clothes, many overweight folks can recall being greeted by a rude or disinterested salesperson. Before a single word has been exchanged, an opinion is forming. Even if it turns out that a particular store doesn't have something in your size, there is an appropriate way for a salesperson to express this fact. The manner in which an obese person can be told that they don't have a particular size need not be any different than how a tall person is told, but generally it isn't. Don't allow it! If the salesperson seems reluctant to give her full effort, indicate that you expect to be treated the same as any other customer. If after repeated efforts to find something you are unable, then you will gladly concede. Don't be funny and make jokes about it, and certainly don't be a doormat and simply head for the exit. If you see yourself as the bitter, angry type, resist the urge to jump down the salesperson's throat. This won't make her want to help you, either.

Insist that they help you in the same way they would help someone who's a size 4. Notice, we're not taking no for an answer (passive) and were not verbally assaulting the salesperson (aggressive), we're simply asking for the same treatment that anyone else would receive (assertive). Whether you're buying a sweater, negotiating the terms of a mortgage, or ordering a decaf latte, it doesn't matter. Any time that you're dealing with other people in this context, you are within your rights to insist that you be treated with respect.

During conversations with friends and family, make efforts to get the focus off of your weight. Most people without weight concerns don't draw attention to the fact that their weight isn't a problem. Neither should you. Imagine talking for the next 20 years about how you used to be heavy! It gets old after a while. Hopefully you'll be hearing some compliments and words of encouragement. Take it all in, but then try to talk about all of the other things going on in life—what you are doing and what you aspire to do—just like everyone else!

Certainly do not tolerate any negative comments about your progress. Everyone thinks they're an expert. Many people will tell you that you should have lost more weight by now. Or they'll be critical if they see you eating a piece of chocolate. In the past, the funny guy would have made a joke about the comment, and the doormat would have said nothing or might have even agreed. The bitter and angry guy would have shot an insult back, perhaps throwing in some colorful language in for good measure.

But your new you will take a different approach. Politely let them know that you and your surgeon (the two true experts) agree that things are going as they should and that you appreciate their concern. If you wish, you can then let them know how they could be more supportive. If people make these silly comments because they are ineffectively trying to help, your job is to educate them as to what they can say or do to be helpful.

From time to time you'll encounter an individual who doesn't seem to be championing your cause. Perhaps this person is threatened by your weight loss. Maybe they don't like the fact that you're now in the limelight and they want to knock you down a peg. Remember the *show stealer* from chapter 14? Let them assertively know that you won't stand for it. Take them aside, if possible, and inform them that their comments are upsetting and unwarranted and that you would like them to stop. Maybe they didn't even realize they were saying things that you found upsetting. It's your duty to let them know.

If this diplomatic approach does not work, do not become aggressive. Be increasingly assertive. Make a statement that is even more forceful. Or when they say things in the company of others, immediately let them know that you find their comments to be inappropriate and would like them to stop. They will actually be embarrassing themselves, and that should do the trick.

If the damaging critique doesn't seem to stop, even in the face of your increased assertiveness, you'll need to question whether you want to continue the relationship. Unfortunately, after weight loss surgery many people learn that those they thought were friends were not such good friends after all.

Going Forward

As you become more comfortable learning how to be assertive in these initial situations, you'll want to seek out new opportunities where you can experiment and flex your assertiveness muscles. Make it a point to practice these skills as often as possible. The world does a fine job of putting us in situations where we need to express ourselves and make our wishes known. Don't shy away!

As you master verbal assertiveness, make it a point to practice some of the more subtle nonverbal forms of assertive communication. Work on increasing your eye contact and maintaining a more assertive posture—no slouching! Face people when you speak to them, rather than angling off to the side. The use of hand gestures is often a sign of assertiveness; practice these, as well. With continued effort you'll no longer feel as if you are practicing or acting like an assertive person. You will *become* an assertive person!

17

Telling Others

S HOULD I TELL PEOPLE ABOUT my weight loss surgery? We briefly
touched on this question in chapter 6. Prior to surgery, most
of my patients tell only the handful of people they believed
they had to tell, both to gather their opinions as well as to ensure that
they had their support.

After surgery, the decision regarding whom to tell is a bit different. You are certainly under no obligation to tell anyone. After all,
it's your own, private medical situation. But the changes that weight
loss surgery brings are quite dramatic and very noticeable to even
the most casual observer. So it's only natural that you would ask this
question. Some of these thoughts may be on your mind:

"What will people think of me for having had surgery?"

"If my friends or loved ones find out that I had surgery,
would they be angry with me for not telling them sooner?"

"If I don't tell, wouldn't people notice that I'm eating differently?"

"What if I tell people about the surgery and then I regain

the weight? I would be so humiliated!"

These questions all conjure up considerable anxiety. Try to keep this anxiety from making the decision for you. For the most part, my experience is that loved ones come around to support your decision to have surgery whether you tell them before or after the procedure. In addition, when you lose weight and feel good about yourself, experience tells me that most people are far less concerned about the critical opinions of others.

Whom To Tell?

Whom are you going to tell first? The answer to this question really depends on your goals for disclosure. Why are you telling anyone, anyway? The usual answer is support and encouragement. Of course, you'll also want to tell folks whose opinions you value. When you use these two goals to define whom to tell, the number of folks dwindles pretty quickly. It's probably a short list, and it should be. In fact, many of the people on your list already know because you've already consulted them before having the surgery.

Whom are you going to tell next? As you broaden your disclosure, again keep in mind your two goals: support and valued opinions. You naturally don't want to share with people who couldn't care less or who might fling destructive commentary. So at this point you'll want to extend your revelations to those you encounter the most, like your close coworkers and other acquaintances. In some cases they'll ask you first, and that's okay.

Will you tell the world? In this age of ubiquitous electronic communication, people already know much more about you than they did only a generation ago. Regardless of whether you've ever even been online, there are probably profiles about you on the Internet that you don't even know about. So it's not unusual for you to wonder whether you should disclose your surgery through your already established routine online social networking. Before you login and wallpaper your personal Web site with all those before and after photographs, please stop for a moment and remember those two disclosure goals: support and valued opinions. If you go public, will those who see you really have the capacity to provide you with support? Do they really even know you? Will they care? Be mindful and careful before you post anything online.

You may think that posting your story online will help many others who are struggling with obesity and weight loss. That may be the case. But before you go out and save the world, consider your own support first. Like with those airplane oxygen masks, put yours on first before you tend to those around you. Focus on those few people that you really value and need in your inner circle. All of the other folks can wait for later, if ever.

How To Tell?

Now that you know *whom* to tell, let's explore *how* to tell. I've never been a big fan of making a long drawn out script of what to say. It's probably a good idea to jot down a few thoughts, but nothing too formal. Overdoing it is going to make you anxious about sticking to a script.

Keep it simple: "You're a really important person to me and I want you to be a part of this big change that I'm making in my life," or "I've made a major decision and I want to share it with you." Again, don't script it too much. Remember that you are sharing your thoughts with friends and loved ones, and they are the folks in your life who are the most likely to be sympathetic and understanding.

A good approach might be to recall how you told those few people before you had surgery. What did you tell them? How did they respond? Odds are you've involved them in the process early on, before you were sure of your decision. Therefore, your anxiety was minimal because you hadn't yet fully committed to the idea.

Now you're on the other side of surgery. It's already done! You're not telling someone to get an opinion and support on having the surgery. You're telling them because you value them in your life and want them to be a part of a fantastic change you've made. I'd like you to think of your decision to disclose as bestowing an honor: I value you in my life so much that I'm giving you the honor of knowing about a major change that I've made. You're not really asking them something; you're giving them something.

When To Tell?

When to disclose your weight loss surgery is perhaps less important than to *whom* and *how*, but timing occasionally comes into play. Your closest confidants already know. But for your broader social network, here is one simple approach: Many of my patients decide to tell others when officially asked, "What did you do to lose weight?" A number of my patients tell me that they don't really want to lie. So if a person they like and value asks them the big question, they just tell the truth.

If you have a close group of friends, there is a good chance they will notice when you've lost 25 pounds or so. You might be able to initially deflect the question by saying you're on a diet. But when 25 pounds becomes 50 or more, the diet story becomes a harder sell. Every once in a while, a patient tells me that a friend or family member was upset that they weren't told sooner. But most people recognize that it's a very personal decision and don't really become that upset. Most also have a sense of the closeness of their relationship to you. It is uncommon and would be a bit bizarre if a friend who you see or speak to less than once in a great while was offended that they were not in the inner sanctum of those you chose to tell sooner.

Delaying the decision by trying to wait for "the right moment" could eventually increase your anxiety. Without question, if you wait until you've lost 75 pounds or more and don't tell, or even go so far as to deny that you've had surgery, some people will start to talk. They'll start to observe your eating habits to see if they can figure it out for themselves. Some people can get quite catty, both because they're curious and maybe even a bit jealous.

Why Aren't You Telling?

I'm not going to suggest that you *should* be telling anyone and everyone, but let me play devil's advocate for a moment. Are you not telling because you're embarrassed? Are you not telling because you think you cheated or took the easy way out by having surgery? I'm making an issue of this point because I want you to be comfortable with the choice you've made. You need to feel proud about your decision.

For a moment, forget what you tell others. To truly move forward with your life, you need to feel comfortable first with what you tell *yourself*. What you say to yourself greatly influences your willingness to tell others. Go back and review how you made this decision to have surgery for yourself. Why did you decide to have surgery? Think about this for a while and become comfortable with the steps that led you to this decision. You knew there was no other rational way to lose that much weight. You knew you had already tried almost everything else. You knew your health was in jeopardy and you were tired of missing out on all that life has to offer. This is nothing to be embarrassed about! And as anyone who has had surgery can tell you, surgery is hardly "the easy road."

Let's take this discussion a step further. Let's say that it was possible that you could have lost all the weight through diet and exercise if you just tried a little harder. In fact, there are some people who do it, the ones you see on daytime talk shows or on late night infomercials for the wonder product de jour. Here's my question to you: Why must it say something negative about you simply because you chose what *may* have been an easier or more reliable path to achieve lasting weight loss? What's wrong with trying to do something an easier way? How is this cheating?

Millions of people have tried a variety of medications to control their appetite and lose weight. Was that cheating? While we're at it, isn't exercise cheating? Why not just eat less and not rely upon treadmills to burn off excess calories? Why not just control your calorie intake so there are no excess calories? Isn't using a dishwasher or a washing machine cheating? Why can't you wash your own clothes or dishes by hand? You can see where this argument is going.

There is nothing wrong with using a tool to help make behavior change easier. It's only when the easier road now causes greater problems later that there is a problem. There is no nobility in failing at one method (dieting) over and over and over again. Finding another way—a better way—is a sign of intelligence, not laziness or failure.

If you review the steps you took to reach surgery, and you're truly comfortable with your decision, you will care far less about what others think whether you decide to tell them. You made a decision to address a significant health concern and improve your quality of life.

It was a wise decision. Be proud of the fact that you had the courage to take advantage of a method that truly works to help address a formidable health problem. Learn to be comfortable demonstrating that pride to others. And remember: It isn't necessary for you to tell everyone of your decision, just those whom you want to tell and those who you think will support your continued journey.

Part V
Dealing With Myself

A central part of the weight loss surgery journey is adapting to a slimmer and healthier body. But after years of living with the hurtful insinuation and attacks of others, it's sometimes hard to shake the internalized destructive thoughts and feelings that go along with that old body. Life after surgery requires you to come to terms with not only a new body, but also a new identity, with changing feelings, thoughts, and behaviors. We explore how to deal with depression, which can set you back. And we learn new tools to enhance your self-esteem, which can move you forward. Ultimately, we help define the new you.

18

Developing a Positive Self-Image

S O YOU'VE HAD WEIGHT LOSS surgery and you're losing weight. Perhaps you've even reached your weight loss goal. But what about your self-image and body image goals? Do you feel the way you wanted to feel about your body and yourself now that you're thinner? Is it what you expected?

It's unfortunate that many folks who have had weight loss surgery and have lost considerable weight find that they don't feel as good about their body or themselves as they thought they would. Changing your opinion about the person you see in the mirror often requires more than just losing weight. As you already know from earlier chapters, it's easier to get rid of *fat body* than *fat brain*. Let's discuss why this is so, and learn what can be done about it.

Self-Image, Self-Worth, Self-Esteem and Body Image

It's important to distinguish between self-image and body image. Self-image is the larger category, so let's begin there. *Self-image* is an assessment of what you think about yourself—of how you see yourself, your value, or your worth. You likely have many different self-images, one for each unique role you play in life. And each self-image is like one slice of a larger pie. Some example of these slices include your work self, your parenting self, your athletic self, and so on.

When you add up all of the separate slices of your self-image, the total is often what we call your *self-worth*. It's as if we score or rank ourselves on each of these roles and total it up to derive an overall score or "worth." Unfortunately, many people convert the score into a pass–fail system. I'm good or I'm bad. I'm a winner or I'm a loser. Of course it's not quite that simple.

Self-worth and self-image are a bit different. Self-image answers the question: Who am I? Self-worth answers the question: What do I think of myself? Self-worth is synonymous with *self-esteem* in that both terms refer to an assessment of your overall worth or value. There are numerous pitfalls in coming up with an accurate gauge of both self-image and self-worth. Some people assess their self-worth or overall goodness or badness based upon their income, the type of car they drive, the number of dollars they've donated, or the type of parties they get invited to. Some people assess their self-worth based upon the size of jeans they wear.

Body image is how we feel about our body and our appearance, and represents only one slice of a person's entire self-image. Unfortunately, too many folks see self-image and body image as the same thing. In assessing her self-image, one woman said to me, "I'm fat, and that's that." To this woman, as long as she was fat, there was nothing further to discuss. The fact that she had numerous successes in other areas of her life and was well loved by friends and family was almost irrelevant. Her jeans size wasn't what it should be and that's what was most important to her. It might sound ridiculous when I put it this way, but I'm guessing that you sometimes endorse this type of thinking yourself.

Body Image Does Not Equal Self-Image

How in the world did weight become so all-encompassing and all-important in the definitions of ourselves? Why are millions of stories in magazines, newspapers, and television dedicated to obesity every single year? Why do people link such a huge portion of their self-image to their waist or dress size? The reasons are complex, but

I suspect a large contributor to this equation is the huge value our society places on appearance and beauty. It's drilled into our heads: If you look good, you feel good. True, dressing sharp may make you may feel good. But it's a huge leap to bounce from a single perception about your body to a judgment of your entire self-image.

To conclude that your self-image is equal to what you see in the mirror is a gross overgeneralization—and just plain wrong! But that's exactly what many people do. Likening your weight or your dress size to your self-worth is a serious mistake, and this is a hard lesson to learn as you lose weight. You reach the weight loss goal and now have your desired jeans size, but fail to achieve the goal of self-acceptance and improved self-worth. What went wrong?

Part of the problem is that some folks may lose sight of the reality that losing weight after surgery is only one piece of improving your self-image. Some people get so locked into numeric objectives like a particular weight or a particular pants size that they lose sight of the real reasons they wanted to lose weight: To improve their health, functioning and quality of life. One of the peculiarities about obesity in our society is just how obsessed people are with weight. Sure, obesity is unhealthy and viewed by many as being unattractive. But it is still only one aspect of who you are.

Understandably, many people tell me that they want to lose weight so they can like themselves more or feel better about themselves. To be fair, most people do enjoy a significant bounce in self-worth and acceptance after losing weight. But a shrinking number on a scale alone doesn't ensure that self-worth will improve. Why? Because self-image evolves over time. A person's self-image is either nurtured or abused, by others and ourselves, over the course of many years. And self-image is greatly affected by many factors such as family history, gender and cultural background. It is a complex feature of your total identity. To bank your entire self-image on one number (a size or a weight) is quite ludicrous.

Believe it or not, not everyone with a diminished body image has a poor self-image. I have had the pleasure of meeting many obese people who recognize size as only one element of their identity. They were not happy with their weight, but refused to allow it to define who they were and what they could achieve. This is actually the first step in moving your self-esteem in a more positive direction: Recognize that body image is only one slice of your self-image.

Big Guy versus Big Girl

Societal expectations play a significant role in the development of self-image. Especially relevant is gender, where there are real differences between how overweight men and women are viewed and ultimately evaluated by others. And these differing societal perceptions and evaluations affect the individual: You begin to see yourself as the world sees you.

It appears that most men support the idea that you can be overweight and still like yourself. In our American culture, there are far fewer demands placed on men to be thin, relative to women. Society more readily accepts overweight men than women. As a result, men generally don't experience the self-loathing that women do. Prior to surgery, I rarely hear a man tell me that he avoids social interaction or intimate relationships because he is obese. There is room in American culture for the *big guy*. It's perfectly okay to be a big burly football player.

Conversely, I rarely hear a woman tell me that her weight has not affected her social or intimate life in some negative way. Apparently, there is no room in our society for the *big girl*. It's completely unacceptable to be a big burly cheerleader. So it seems that a woman's weight and size are more likely to define a woman than a man.

Believing What Isn't True

As others tell us over and over that our weight defines us, we start to believe them. And then we repeat the same message to ourselves, blossoming into a *self-fulfilling prophecy*. No matter how harshly we are judged by our families and society, it is often no match for how critical we are of ourselves. Regrettably, we are often our own worst critics. Let me share an example.

> One of my post-surgical weight loss patients (let's call her Rachel) told me that she always thought of herself as a "fat, ugly, dumb, slob." She admitted that no one ever called her any of these names; she did it to herself. Whenever someone looked at her, if an interview went poorly, or if a man

failed to return her phone call, in her mind it was because she was a Fat, Ugly, Dumb, Slob (FUDS).

I pointed out to Rachel that she didn't think of herself as "Rachel." She thought of herself as "FUDS." And despite the fact that weight was melting off with each passing week after surgery, she still thought of herself as FUDS. It was hard for her to separate being fat from being ugly and a slob. And despite the fact that she was a bright woman, she labeled herself as dumb.

It was clear that over the past 20 years Rachel had equated her self-worth with her weight, and her identity had evolved into FUDS. Even though her weight was diminishing rapidly, the label stuck. No single improvement on the bathroom scale could kill FUDS. *Fat body* was retreating fast, but *fat brain* was slow to catch up. More work was needed.

Obese people often endure a great deal of abuse (or neglect) from others. Soon they internalize this abuse and begin to recite it to themselves, actually believing that the destructive critique is actually true. This leads them to avoid and withdraw from others in a variety of ways. Overweight people often feel highly self-conscious, and are on high alert for anything that confirms their self-loathing. When they hear something that even mildly insinuates "you're fat," many will recoil. They stop socializing, withdraw, and become timid or passive. The diminished self-worth is soon communicated back to the world, and often they don't even recognize that it's happening. Nonverbal behavior says it all, like avoiding eye contact, looking down, slouching, and maintaining a closed or tense posture. It's a language that communicates: "I'm no good."

Even after you've lost a significant amount of weight, others may continue to respond to you awkwardly. This no longer occurs because of your weight, but because you're continuing to act as if you're not worthy of their attention. They're responding to your residual poor self-image, which is the fat brain that has yet to catch up with the thinning body. With such continued social rejection, you use it as confirmation that you're still no good, even as a thinner person, and berate yourself further. It becomes a self-defeating downward spiral. How can this be stopped?

Changing Your Thoughts

Changing your self-image involves making a concerted effort to treat yourself with respect, and insist that others do, as well. It involves changing your self-talk as well as your behaviors. What is self-talk you ask? *Self-talk* is what we tell ourselves in our head, kind of like thinking. But it's a self-directed form of thinking where we are essentially talking to ourselves.

Do you remember that classic story of *The Little Engine That Could* by Watty Piper? Recall that the engine kept repeating "I think I can, I think I can." That positive self-talk was largely responsible for the little engine making his way up and over the big hill. What you tell yourself about yourself and the world around you is hugely important in how you proceed and succeed in the world. Perhaps my favorite example of this was a comment made by the Jedi Master Yoda to the young apprentice Luke Skywalker in the second *Star Wars* film, *The Empire Strikes Back.* Yoda used the power of the force to lift Luke's star fighter out of a swamp and across the sky to a more secure location after Luke failed to do so himself. Upon seeing Yoda perform this action, Luke replied, "I don't believe it!" Yoda responded, "That is why you fail." How you think is everything. Changing your self-talk is crucial.

Developing new self-talk requires making consistent efforts to adopt a rational and accurate perception of yourself, and to be supportive of yourself as you make changes. Thinking of yourself as "FUDS" is a good example of being irrational and unsupportive. Improving your self-image involves reintroducing you to yourself, and relearning who you are. This takes practice, time and effort, so be patient. But also don't give up. Your surgery helped you reduce *fat body.* Now it's time for you to work on reducing *fat brain.*

A great guidepost in this process is to ask yourself how you would advise a friend. Isn't it fascinating how we are so much better at being inspiring and encouraging to others compared to ourselves? You would certainly tell a friend who had weight loss surgery how great she looks and compliment her on all her progress. You'd be supportive of your friend during this process as she negotiates her successes and setbacks. You'd tell her to keep trying and you'd shoot down her self-deprecating and self-defeating comments. Why not extend that same kind and nurturing treatment to yourself?

Changing Your Behaviors

In addition to initiating and incorporating new elements of self-talk into your repertoire, making changes in your behaviors is equally essential. These behavior changes involve learning and actively practicing new skills. You don't have to wait until you *feel* more confident with yourself to start *acting* more comfortable with yourself. Sounds funny, doesn't it? Why are we so insistent that changes in feelings must come first?

Here is the basic concept: If you want to become a thinner, more self-assured and confident person, start behaving how you believe thin, self-assured, confident people act. Observe those friends or others of an appropriate weight who seem to have that confident vibe or aura about them. Make a list of all of the obvious and subtle behaviors that communicate self-confidence and try them out. Here are some places to start:

- ✓ Improve your posture.
- ✓ Make better eye contact.
- ✓ Wear more flattering clothing instead of baggy, shapeless outfits.
- ✓ Speak positively about yourself in conversation, and stop self-deprecating comments.
- ✓ Smile.
- ✓ Get into the mix of conversation.
- ✓ Offer your opinion.

If you're having difficulty identifying some of these behaviors, ask a close friend or two to tell you what they see you doing that communicates a poor self-image. It's very likely that this process of "fake it 'till you make it" will feel awkward or phony at first. Don't be concerned with how it feels right now. With time you'll become more comfortable with these new behaviors, and the good feelings will soon follow.

A Work in Progress

Improving your self-image is not a weekend project, but rather a process that will take months if not years. And it's never truly complete. We're always evolving throughout our lives, striving for gradual self-improvement, and that's a good thing.

If you are yearning for more advice and direction about improving how you feel about yourself, chapter 20 provides some tips to get you started. However a complete self-esteem makeover is beyond the scope of this book. So you might want to take a look at Glenn Schiraldi's *Self-Esteem Workbook*, referenced in appendix C.

With effort and persistence it is absolutely possible to achieve what may have been one of your true purposes in having weight loss surgery: To love your body *and* love yourself.

19

Depression After Weight Loss Surgery

BEFORE WE TRY TO UNDERSTAND how depression might be related to weight loss surgery, it's important for us to have a clear definition of depression. When most lay people use the word depression, what they really mean is feeling sad or upset. I refer to this as *little-d depression*. Used in this way, being depressed refers to a temporary negative mood state. This type of depression can last a few days and affects some aspects of the person's functioning. These negative moods are a normal and expected part of life. We all experience little-d depression from time to time.

The depression of greater concern is the type that is more enduring and has more of an effect on a person's functioning. This type of depression is what I call *big-D depression*. With big-D depression, the symptoms are more significant and longer lasting. The term used to describe big-D in the psychological literature is Major Depression. When someone is experiencing an episode of Major Depression, they are experiencing a depressed mood almost every day for at least two weeks, and there is usually a significantly diminished interest or pleasure in most, if not all, activities. So the person is not just bummed out about one or two things, but about nearly everything.

Furthermore, when someone is experiencing Major Depression, they don't just feel extremely sad. Several of the following additional symptoms are present almost every day for at least two weeks: significant changes in appetite, a lack of energy, a noticeable slowdown or difficulty in movement, feelings of worthlessness or excessive guilt, difficulty concentrating, significant changes in sleep patterns by sleeping notably more or less than usual, and recurrent thoughts of death or suicide. These symptoms cause clinically significant distress or impairment in social, occupational, or other important areas of functioning. Plus, these symptoms cannot be explained by the direct effects of a medication, drug or medical problem, and are not a consequence of bereavement, such as after the loss of a loved one. To meet the official criteria for a Major Depressive Episode, one must have five or more of these symptoms happening rather continuously for a minimum of two weeks, and those symptoms must cause considerable distress and adversely affect the person's functioning. The severity of a Major Depressive Episode can range from mild, when an individual has just enough symptoms to meet the criteria for diagnosis, to severe, where the individual has almost all of the symptoms listed above.

As you can see, Major Depression is *very* different from what most folks call depression. Big-D depression represents not only a change in how you feel, but how you act and function, as well. You will no doubt now think twice before you tell your friend how "depressed" you are that the Yankees lost or that your boyfriend didn't call last night.

What's Depression Like After Weight Loss Surgery?

Weight loss surgery requires a great number of behavioral changes, some of which cause temporary emotional discomfort. It's hard to change what you're eating and difficult to go without some of the foods you like. It's strange to try and chew your food 25 times before swallowing. Soon after surgery, it can be awkward to go to restaurants or to attend affairs that involve eating where you simply cannot eat the way you used to. Many patients have confided that they initially felt awkward, uncomfortable and even a bit unhappy at these events. However, after a time, most indicate that they were able to make the necessary adjustments so that they could better enjoy these situations. This type of little-d depression is important to discuss and prepare for, but it does not necessitate calling out the cavalry.

Most folks you hear being described as depressed following weight loss surgery are experiencing little-d, not big-D. They may be experiencing a few of these symptoms for more than two weeks, but probably not five or more of them. Most weight loss surgery patients experience ups and downs in dealing with the transitions and challenges of having surgery and coping with all its associated changes.

Of course, it is certainly possible that some folks experience a few symptoms of big-D, or perhaps they truly do meet the criteria for Major Depression. If this happens, concern and attention are certainly warranted. In my experience, the symptoms of big-D most commonly reported following weight loss surgery include depressed mood, diminished interest in some activities, and feelings of worthlessness. Decreased appetite and weight loss are also probably occurring, but this is likely because of the surgery, not because of depression. Nonetheless, it's important to not ignore something more severe:

> If you are experiencing a number of these big-D symptoms, the most important step is to acknowledge that these symptoms are occurring, and that they are not to be ignored or tolerated. Seek professional help as soon as possible.

This may seem rather obvious. However, it's quite common for someone to ignore their distress for a long period of time and only begin to address it after more damage has been done. People unfortunately do this with medical problems as well, and the consequences of waiting can be tragic. If you or a loved one is experiencing symptoms of big-D depression, there are a variety of treatment options available, including individual and group counseling with a mental health professional, support groups, or antidepressant medication. You can learn more about each of these options and more in appendix A.

The Controversy

Not to long ago, a controversy exploded in the media regarding the link between weight loss surgery and depression. Indeed, many reports in the media suggested that weight loss surgery actually *caused* depression, and even suicide. Was this true? Could big-D depression be a major side effect of weight loss surgery?

To gain some perspective on this issue, it is helpful to turn back the clock to when weight loss surgery first began receiving increased media attention. At that time, almost every news story and daytime talk show host delighted in trotting successful patients out onto the stage, showing their before and after pictures, and portraying surgery as nothing short of a miracle. These shows rarely discussed the hard work the patients went through to achieve such results. They only showed the nightmare of morbid obesity before, and the happier ending after, but not the journey in between.

Suddenly, in typical media fashion, surgery was being portrayed as not only somewhat less than miraculous, but even fatal! Most unfortunate is that the media's highlighting of some of the less common consequences of weight loss surgery is frightening the very people that the surgery would most benefit. So prevalent was this concern about depression that a growing number of patients expressed anxiety about becoming depressed after losing weight during my initial meeting with them. Patients told me that they are concerned that they "won't be as funny" or that they will "lose their spark" or "become a hermit" when they "can't eat" and become thinner. From all the media hype, you could easily be led to believe that depression following weight loss surgery is quite common. This cause for concern was at least worthy of closer inspection.

As a child, I often took what others said to be the truth. Many kids do; it's normal at a young age. But my mother used to remind me all the time, "Take it from where it comes, and with a grain of salt." In the case of weight loss surgery, much of the information on its potential adverse consequences comes from anecdotal patient stories portrayed and sometimes exaggerated by the news media.

The problem with anecdotal stories is that while they can be quite compelling, they often fail to give the entire picture. We see the person telling their story in their current tragic state, and its emotional impact strikes a chord in us. However, we don't know about the person's history and we're only getting their version of events. Yes, I have treated individual patients who experienced symptoms of depression following weight loss surgery. But they represent only a handful of people out of the hundreds of successful weight loss surgery patients that I've also seen. Additionally, among those patients who did experience depression, it was most often mild and temporary.

When it comes to the news media, you *really* need to "take it from where it comes, and with a grain of salt." I've watched several episodes of various talk shows and have seen Internet video clips that highlight marital breakups, substance abuse, family discord, depression and other negative consequences attributed to weight loss surgery. All of this drama is great for ratings, but does a disservice to people who are watching these shows in search of accurate and balanced information on weight loss surgery. While there may have been an association between weight loss surgery and these unfortunate outcomes for the people on these shows, saying that the surgery *caused* such outcomes is often a reach.

As a psychologist working in the area of weight loss surgery for several years, I can attest that while these consequences can and do happen after surgery, they are not common. Plus they are not likely a direct consequence of the surgery, but rather of the emotional changes that occur as a result of making the various behavioral changes necessitated by weight loss surgery. Strict adherence to a diet would likely be no different than weight loss surgery.

The media has a penchant for hyping the latest medical procedure as miraculous, only later to delight in showing all of its possible drawbacks. We've seen it with celebrity status in chapter 14, and we see it here, as well: Build it up—tear it down. Highlighting the extremes of miraculous success and disastrous consequences do wonders for viewership and ratings. Think about it: A show that highlighted only moderate success stories or modest difficulties about weight loss surgery wouldn't attract viewers. But "Weight Loss Surgery Nightmare!" or "Surgery Saved My Life!" gets your attention and implores you to tune in. The moral of the story is that when you want to conduct research on something, daytime talk shows and personal online videos should not be high on your list of reliable places to gather information.

So what's the truth about the association between depression and weight loss surgery? The overwhelming majority of patients that I have seen do *not* experience a clinically significant depression following weight loss surgery. Those who do have depressive symptoms after surgery do not have symptoms of the severity that warrant coverage on daytime talk shows. As someone who has had weight loss surgery, you know the whole story. If you're like most of my patients, you're gratified for having made the decision to have surgery. You have a rational view of surgery as being quite helpful, but not miraculous. You've had good days and some bad days. And you understand all of the hard work involved in adjusting to the changes required for success.

What's Unique About Depression After Weight Loss Surgery?

Everyone knows what depression feels like. But when it derives from the long history of struggle with obesity, as well as all the changes that come after weight loss surgery, it takes on a unique character. Here are some of the comments I've heard from my patients over the years, all of which paint one shade or another of depression. Perhaps you'll recognize some of yourself in these experiences of little-d or big-D after weight loss surgery:

"I don't feel as relaxed at social gatherings without the food. I almost feel naked."

"I sometimes feel so angry that I can't eat some of the things I want. At times I'd rather not even go to a party than to be faced with foods that I can't eat."

"As I've lost more and more weight, I find at times I don't even recognize myself."

"I feel so sad and angry with myself for all the years I spent trapped in that obese body. How did I let myself get that way?"

"Now that I've lost the weight, everyone is pressuring me to do things: Get a new job, start dating, go shopping, whatever. I feel overwhelmed by all of it!"

"When people make positive comments about how much better I now look and how much more confident I now seem, I can't help but wonder what they must have thought of me *before* I lost all of the weight."

"In some strange way, life was simple before surgery. All I ever thought about was losing weight. Now that I've lost the weight I don't know what I should be focusing on. It's like I'm lost in my own life."

"In some ways, I don't even know who I am anymore."

"I feel like I'm always on display. I'm tired of people asking me how much weight I've lost."

"I've lost all this weight and things really aren't that much different. I'm just thinner now. I was hoping for more."

"The only thing that's different is that losing weight is no longer on my to do list."

"Nobody understands what I'm going through. I feel so alone."

"I'm obviously thrilled about losing the weight, but now I have all of this excess skin. I thought I'd feel more confident about my body, but I still can't imagine allowing anyone to see me this way."

I sincerely hope that you're saying to yourself, Wow, I don't have it that bad! If you read these comments and can hear yourself saying some of these things, I want you to understand that you're not alone and that brighter days are ahead. Some of these comments bring up issues that I've discussed in previous chapters, so it might be worthwhile going back for a second read. Then come back here to look more closely at why feelings of depression develop following weight loss surgery.

Why Might Depression Occur After Weight Loss Surgery?
The simple answer to this question is that there is no simple answer. Depression happens for a myriad of reasons, even in the unique situation after weight loss surgery. Let's explore some of those reasons.

1. Weight loss surgery requires making a number of changes. Change can be stressful, and prolonged stress can lead to depression.
Over the years, much research has been dedicated to the study of stress. In today's society, the stress of day-to-day life is getting worse and the effects of stress are garnering a great deal of attention. One popular theory is that change, itself, causes stress. Many years ago, a popular stress scale was created that measured the extent of someone's level of stress by what were called "life change units." The researchers proposed that the greater the number and severity of life changes an individual was experiencing, the greater the stress. Of note was the fact that changes involving positive events, such as getting married, the birth of a child, or a promotion at work also caused stress. Although positive, these events still result in significant changes in one's daily functioning and are therefore considered stressful.

Human beings are creatures of habit. We tend to function best when there is a routine and some structure to our lives. People tend to wake up at the same time each day, drive to work using the same route, buy the same products at the supermarket, eat in the same restaurants, and so on. Once a ritual is formed, we're reluctant to change. It's as though our brain is trying to make life easier for us.

Consider the toothpaste you use. It's probably either Crest or Colgate, the two big brands in the United States. If you were to ask yourself why you buy the brand you buy, you'd probably come up with some thoughtful and sensible reason. But the truth is that you probably buy Crest because you've *always* bought Crest. Odds are that your parents bought Crest, as well. When a behavior or a habit becomes part of our routine, we tend to stick with it. Random, spontaneous change is not the norm for most people. It's like buying a different brand of toothpaste every week—maybe worse.

Weight loss surgery requires you to make a number of changes. First of all, you have to eat differently. You have to chew differently. You may have to eat different foods. Many things about what you eat, where you eat, when you eat and how you eat will be changing. If change equals stress, then that's a lot of stress! And if stress sometimes leads to depression, you can see where I'm going with this.

After weight loss surgery, however, it's not all gloom and doom. The stress and consequent depression usually subside. A new routine settles in. After a few months, you probably will have adjusted to most of the eating and food-related changes. With the passing of several months to a year, you'll likely know what to order in a restaurant or at a catered affair. You'll know how many times to chew your favorite food for it to go down comfortably. This is good progress.

Of course, your eating habits involve only one facet of adjustment after weight loss surgery. You'll also need to contend with all the emotional changes you experience, and in how others respond to you. Losing 100 pounds (or thereabouts) is no trivial event. It's a major life change. At the very least, your body's physical changes are quite radical. It's likely that you've noticed changes in the way you behave, as well. You probably feel differently about yourself and your body. The manner in which people interact with you has probably changed. There are possibly more complements. You're being paid greater attention. Many of these changes are positive, but they can still cause stress.

Perhaps you've noticed that you've changed the way you interact and feel around others. Initially, these changes can be quite stressful, and if there have been difficulties in adjusting to all of this, feelings of depression can ensue. You may feel uncomfortable, sad, or anxious regarding some of these changes. Much of this is normal. Just like the changes you made in your eating habits, once time has passed and you've settled into your new stable routine, and once you've grown accustomed to the changes in the way you feel along with how others interact with you, the depressive feelings will likely diminish. If they don't, you might need to take some of those extra steps to address the depression that we discussed earlier in this chapter.

2. My identity is different. Sometimes I don't recognize myself.

Think back to just how many years you went through life as a morbidly obese person. Was it ten years, 20 years? Thirty or 40 years? For many folks who struggle with morbid obesity, their weight is more than a physical description; it's a personality description, as well. If you've been overweight since childhood, you've probably seen your weight as an intrinsic part of your identity. Now that you're thinner, you've changed. Although it may appear that only your weight has changed, it's really so much more.

Many patients admit that they don't recognize themselves anymore. The changes in the way they behave and the way others are behaving towards them are so dramatic that they're not sure how to respond. One woman went so far as to say, "I don't feel like a thinner version of myself. I feel like a different person. It's as if I woke up one morning and was a different race." This obviously would be quite stressful, to not recognize yourself in your own body.

Developing a new identity after weight loss surgery is all part of leaving *fat brain* behind. Part of fat brain involves thinking like a person who's still obese, and you already know that your *fat body* will arrive well ahead of your fat brain. Revisit chapters 14, 16 and 18 to refresh your memory about this distinction. Part of your fat brain identity may have included you seeing yourself as the *funny guy*, the *doormat*, or the bitter and angry *loner*. Chapter 16 explored these three unproductive identities, and all three can make you prone to depression.

Are you wondering how a funny guy could possibly be prone to depression? Well, weight loss surgery essentially stole his punch line. Now that the funny guy is thinner, making self-deprecating jokes about weight just doesn't work anymore. He's no longer overweight. The funny guy can no longer make funny fat jokes, so he might feel strange in his new non-comedic role. It's understandable that he might be searching for a new identity.

In fact, this is something I hear from time to time from patients considering surgery: "I knew a guy who used to be a riot! But after he had surgery he wasn't as funny anymore. It's like he lost his sense of humor or something. Will this happen to me?" He probably didn't lose his sense of humor; he just couldn't use his weight as the subject of his jokes anymore. He also may have lost a bit of his sense of self. He's not the same guy as he was 100 pounds ago and he may need some time to adjust to changes in how he feels about himself as well as how others interact with him.

This change in your overall view of yourself will take some time to get used to. During the time you are adjusting, you'll likely experience the stress of making changes in your behavior. Plus you'll be confronting new and different feelings. There will be some moments of awkwardness and discomfort. If others are treating you a bit like you're a different person, you'll feel strange in your new body. It will take a little time for what is new to become familiar and more comfortable, and ultimately less stressful.

Where can you find solutions to building your new identity after weight loss surgery? One option is to turn back to chapter 16 and learn how to engage in some healthy straight talk (assertiveness). There you can gain some pointers on moving on from the funny guy, the doormat, and the loner. In addition, you can turn forward in the book to chapter 20, where you'll learn more broadly about creating a new identity for yourself.

3. Eating has always been a disproportionate source of joy. Now that I've got to make major changes in my eating, it creates a void.

A number of patients I meet before weight loss surgery indicate that food and the behavior of eating represent one of the true joys in their lives. They look forward to going out to eat. Or they order in much more than most. They clearly recognize that many of their activities revolve around food.

If your primary source of joy is food, cooking or eating, then it makes perfect sense that making major changes in these activities could affect your mood. As we touched on back in chapters 6 and 13, some people are what I lovingly call *foodies*. They watch the food shows. They love to cook. They love to go out to eat. They love to entertain. They love to barbecue. They know where the best restaurants are. They are connoisseurs of all things food.

After weight loss surgery, foodies have a different road to travel than those who became overweight for other reasons. If you loved running but got injured and need to shift to bicycling, you'd probably feel a little-d for a while. If you enjoyed living in New York City but your job transferred you to Chicago, you'd probably become a little-d until you met new people and learned all of the wonderful things about living in your new town. Similarly, if you're a foodie and had weight loss surgery (or tried to diet), it's understandable that you'd go through some little-d until you adjusted to all of the changes from surgery and found yourself *a new normal,* a new balance. Once you establish a new normal where things don't feel as awkward and uncomfortable as before, your little-d will probably subside. You can read more about restoring balance in chapter 21.

4. Eating helps me cope with life's difficulties. Because I can't eat for comfort anymore, I can no longer escape those difficulties.

Many patients are astutely aware of their propensity to eat as a means of comforting themselves from life's challenges. Others are not consciously aware of their feelings, but know that they are soothing themselves with food. Most want this behavior to stop, but really don't know how. We spent a good deal of time exploring this kind of *emotional eating* in chapter 8, and I encourage you to revisit that discussion to refresh your memory. Here we'll more closely examine eating in response to depression.

When it comes to depression after weight loss surgery, most often such patients were depressed *before* surgery. Their greatest concern is that the inability to eat following surgery will remove their most effective method of coping with depression. They're also concerned that the inability to eat will unmask the root of their depression. For these folks, depression is not a consequence of surgery; rather it stems from the inability to eat. Here's a common story:

> I work very hard during the day. I hardly get a second to myself from the moment I arrive at work to the moment I get home. I don't really love my job, but it pays the bills. Sometimes I'm so busy that I don't even get a chance to eat lunch. On the days I do have lunch, it's usually at my desk.

> I really look forward to coming home, getting changed, and eating a large dinner and possibly having some treats afterward. I know this pattern of having a huge dinner and snacking late at night isn't healthy, but by the time I get home, I'm starving! Besides, this is my favorite time of the day, where I can finally relax and unwind. It's one of my few real joys.

This is one of the most frequent stories I hear. In fact, many patients share that prior to surgery they consumed about 90 percent of their daily calories between arriving home from work and bedtime. For these folks, food and eating is their primary means to relax and unwind. They're not unlike the people who pour themselves a Scotch when they get home each night.

The schedule that this person keeps is a major problem in that it crowds out non-eating sources of pleasure. These folks often describe themselves as being "a little depressed" or "sort of depressed" (little-d). They know their routine is a problem, and often they recognize that eating in the evening has become their way to relax in response to their hectic and demanding schedule.

For those who do not enjoy their work or who have minimal social contacts, eating may be their *only* joy. They come home at night, tired, lonely and hungry and a little depressed—a horrible convergence of feelings that is temporarily soothed by eating. For them, life is woefully out of balance. Here is another more serious example of such an experience:

> I don't know how this happened but right now my life is nothing more than going to my boring job and coming home and repeating this five times a week. I don't have many friends right now because I'm just too busy. Every once and a while I go out with some people at work or see my family, but I know it's not enough.
>
> The weekends are the hardest. I'd imagine that most people look forward to weekends when they can relax and spend time with their friends or families. But for me the weekend is hell. I just sit at home with not much to do. I order a pizza and ice cream for myself on Friday nights, like a reward for a hard week I guess. Saturday I run some errands and usually eat out alone, or maybe order in a few

times. Sunday is mostly the same.
I promise myself every Monday that it's going to be different but it never is. It's really depressing.

This person may very well be rolling in the direction of the big-
D. Her destructive eating routine has spilled over to the weekend,
and she pursues very little social contact. The lousy job combined
with the loneliness of social isolation is putting her at greater risk
for serious depression. So the void gets filled with food, a form of
emotional eating.

There's an important connection shared between the two folks
whom I've just described: Both were struggling with depression
(whether little-d or big-D) *before* weight loss surgery. And it's very
likely that they will continue to struggle with depression *after* surgery.
The only difference is that after surgery their favorite strategy for
coping with depression would be significantly curtailed. Suddenly,
that perfect elixir for those nights and weekends would no longer be
available.

These folks have quite a struggle on their hands! In my experience, most knew about their impending struggle before surgery, and
were already wondering how they would wing it after surgery. During their pre-surgical evaluation, many have shared that they rec-
ognized the difficulty of trying to cope without eating when dieting
in the past. Some have told me that these unpleasant feelings were
responsible for relapse from previous diets. They didn't like how they
felt while dieting, so they stopped dieting. One woman confided that
she was so miserable on diets that her husband *asked* her to stop dieting. According to my patient, her husband said that he would rather
her be overweight than irritable and depressed! Some patients have
gone so far as to postpone having surgery until they thought they
were better prepared to deal with this problem. Under such conditions, postponing surgery often makes sense.

If you've had weight loss surgery and you're experiencing some
of these difficulties, they will not go away on their own. If these
stories are carbon copies of your own daily life, it is critical that you
make alterations in the evening ritual. It's not so much that you need
to find something to replace eating, but rather your lifestyle needs an

overhaul. If you believe that you're using food to an excessive degree as a method of self-soothing, you'll need to address this issue as soon as possible. You'll need to make significant changes in your thoughts about food and eating, as well as some of the emotional issues in your life. You'll also need to discover alternative ways of relaxing and unwinding. Here are some pointers to get you started.

Consider that coming home, getting undressed and then eating a big meal and grazing until bedtime is a choice—a bad choice. This ritual has gained habit strength and may seem automatic and out of control to you. But it is not impossible to change. After weight loss surgery, your appetite will be diminished, as will be your capacity to eat. However, if you continue to sit home and isolate yourself, it's likely that your feelings of depression would persist. It's also possible that you'll learn to eat in a manner that diminishes your surgery's ability to help you lose weight by doing things like drinking milk shakes or eating ice cream. Remember the dangers of *meltables* and *dumping syndrome* from chapter 13? By being at home, you're making it harder to lose weight because you remain in the destructive physical and emotional environment that fosters emotional eating.

If you've spent the last ten to 20 years sitting on your couch eating ice cream at night while watching television, the last place in the world you want to be at night after surgery is sitting on that same couch! Instead, come home, change clothes, have a bite to eat, and then get involved in something pleasurable. Activities that require movement or social interaction would be especially desirable. Go to a gym, go for a walk, take a class, volunteer. Virtually anything is better than sitting at home on that couch! Even if you're tired (and everybody is tired), you can't tell me that you don't have enough energy left in the tank to take a ten-minute walk.

Initiating and maintaining these new behaviors will take time. When you begin to make these changes, at first they will feel awkward and uncomfortable because they're not part of your current routine. With time and repetition, these newer activities that you have used to replace eating will come to feel less uncomfortable and perhaps even enjoyable. You'll be able to settle into your new normal. There is little or no hope for any progress if you continue to stay at home and remain socially isolated. By getting out there and doing just about anything *else*, you're greatly improving the odds that you'll be able to turn that depression around.

5. All I ever wanted was to be thinner. I reached my goal and I'm thinner. Now what?
You've stared at this mountain called morbid obesity for years. All you ever wanted was to finally climb the mountain and put it past you. Now that you've lost the weight you find yourself standing at the peak. Congratulations!

As you make your way down the mountain, all giddy and happy with your own success, the cheers from friends start to diminish. People aren't telling you how much different and better you look every day anymore. Your mountaintop success of "thinnerness" is now old news. You're even bored with it, maybe even a little melancholic. Now what?

Many patients share that they feel like a ship that's lost its North Star: "All I ever focused on was losing weight. Now that I've lost weight, I honestly don't know what to do with myself. I never really thought beyond losing the weight." Some people will try to punctuate their weight loss with an accomplishment they know would never have been possible when they were obese, such as running a marathon, hiking canyons, getting a makeover, or buying a new wardrobe. These all represent a great start. But again: What's next?

It takes time to shift gears and look beyond the thinness. Accomplishing a lifelong goal usually results in jubilation and relief: "Whew, I did it!" But it's only a matter of time before your spirit begins to wander again. Without a clear set of goals, sometimes that wanderlust can diminish into disillusionment and depression. But with a good map of your future, you can easily downshift and ride on to the next conquest.

Now that you're thinner, you need to begin the business of constructing that map for the rest of your life. What did you want to accomplish as a thinner person? What were you hoping that being thin would provide? No one can answer these questions for you. Maybe take out a pen and some paper and start a list. If you're feeling confused or disillusioned, such feelings need not derail you. If you're feeling a bit depressed or lost, that's completely understandable. It's okay to not have immediate answers to these questions. In fact, it's better to think about it for a while rather than rushing in to solve it.

It's equally important that you not stuff these questions and feelings under the rug. If you're trying to find your new direction, talk to friends, join a support group, or even consider pursuing psychotherapy. It's important that you make some decisions about where you want your life to go. Life has this uncanny way of moving forward, whether you have a plan or not. Chapter 20 can get you started by exploring some methods to create such a plan. You'll need to create your map with firm goals so that your life can move in a specific and productive direction. If you don't, it will simply meander along. Time waits for no one!

6. How did I let myself get so "fat" in the first place?

From time to time, this question crops up after weight loss surgery. If you've ever asked yourself this question, I want you to consider your faulty thinking for a moment. And I'll be direct: It's as if you can't be happy enough with how well things have gone since surgery, that you have to go searching for something to be upset about.

> "I'm so happy with how things are now. Hmm... Let me see; it can't be all that good. I've got it: Let me dredge up the past and tell myself that I shouldn't have gotten into this mess in the first place!"

Do you remember our discussion about the complexity of obesity in chapters 2 through 5? Go back and refresh your memory, if you need to. While you can take responsibility for some of the behaviors that contributed to your weight gain, it is silly to believe that it could have easily been avoided. By having such thoughts, you are irrationally blaming yourself and self-blame is one of the central irrational thoughts associated with depression.

Do you remember our discussion of the dangerousness of holding irrational beliefs of powerlessness in chapter 9? Erroneously blaming yourself for something that's not your fault can lead to irrational beliefs of powerlessness, hopelessness, and helplessness. And these three beliefs are often central to becoming depressed.

The best antidote for such irrational beliefs is to face them head on. Confront them. Challenge them. Uncover the absurdity of them. You can revisit some good strategies to confront these unwelcome thoughts in chapters 9 and 12. Remember: How you think is everything! Return to chapter 12 to reexamine your old irrational thinking and learn strategies for new rational thinking.

7. Is there more?

It would be irresponsible to not leave the door open to other explanations for depression following weight loss surgery. Sometimes there are biological reasons for depression following weight loss surgery. And significant changes in hormones or other body chemicals can contribute to symptoms of depression.

There are also many personal and social circumstances that are unique to every individual pursuing weight loss surgery, and it's impossible to cover all of them in this book. However, the most common precipitants of depression that I've seen in my own practice have been addressed. And I've attempted to give you a realistic, non-sensational, non-hyped perspective on what depression typically looks like after weight loss surgery.

The Bottom Line

The takeaway message from this chapter is that depression can ensue after weight loss surgery. Generally it is mild. Usually depression occurs as a product of the behavioral and emotional changes that result from losing a dramatic amount of weight, not the surgery itself. If you are experiencing depressive symptoms of a troubling nature, there's absolutely nothing wrong with joining a support group, chatting with others about your story, or participating in some form of counseling to address your concerns. In fact, taking active steps to prevent these concerns before they have a chance to get started is a great idea, a step that may better ensure your success from weight loss surgery.

20

The New Me

I T'S SEVERAL MONTHS OR MORE since you've had weight loss surgery. Hopefully, you've lost a great deal of weight. If you're like most folks, you've probably made a number of adjustments in your eating habits. What you eat and certainly how much you eat has changed. You probably look noticeably different than before your surgery. It's likely that you feel physically better as well, and have noticed some genuine improvements in your ability to function and go about your day. But are you happy with all of these changes? Did you achieve your goals from surgery? Have you developed a new you?

As I described in earlier chapters, some folks essentially remain who they've always been, though now in a thinner body. For these people, the journey is pretty straightforward with few complications. They are thinner and are better able to enjoy their lives. Many can now better enjoy what's already present in their lives. If they're single and have an active social life, perhaps they can start dating a little more and become more active with their friends. If they are married with families, they can now better enjoy spending time with everyone, and can be more active participants with the ones they love.

Other folks encounter a rougher road. For these folks, weight was a major obstacle to leading a decent life before surgery. It was an all-encompassing hindrance to living the kind of life they could only dream of. Now that the weight is under control, they're ready to turn over a new leaf. But they don't have the friends and families for support. They don't have the active social calendar. They're starting from the ground up. Many of these folks may have fit the profile of the bitter and angry *loner* (from chapter 16). They really want to become new people, but they're not sure where to start.

Do-over!

Patients often remind me about the movie *City Slickers* where once Daniel Stern's character was divorced from his wife and realizes that he's lost everything, Billy Crystal's character consoles, "Your life is a do-over." This harks back to your childhood play days: If something went wrong in one of your games (you kicked the soccer ball out of bounds or you reached three strikes in baseball), you could always scream, "Do-over!" And your generous childhood friends would give you a second chance.

Although this might be a bit of an overstatement, many patients feel that after weight loss surgery they need to restart their life, almost like hitting the reset button on a video game. At first this may seem rather daunting, but it doesn't have to be difficult and it can actually be enjoyable. Anytime you undertake a major project—and a do-over of your life would certainly qualify—it helps to recall the parable often attributed to Creighton Abrams that goes something like this: "How does an ant eat an elephant? One bite at a time." (Without even thinking of it, I used a food analogy! Old habits truly die hard.) You've also heard this ancient parable by Lao Tzu: "A journey of a thousand miles begins with one step." These quotations all provide excellent advice. You don't change your entire life in one day. You do it one step at a time. Let's see how.

Cartography 101

Okay, I've hopefully convinced you that you need to move forward gradually—one step at a time. But even before you take that first step, how do you know you're traveling the "right" road? That's easy: Recall from chapter 19 that you need a map or a plan. But where are you going to find such a map? Surely you've checked your car's glove compartment and there's none to be found. Without a map, you're certain to get lost, so you've got to draw your own map. And the way you do this is by creating a list of your life's goals and objectives. That's right: Before you begin to wander down this exciting and incredible new journey after weight loss surgery, I need you to create a good map.

Step 1: List your goals.

Don't worry that you never took a cartography course. And don't bother reaching for that GPS unit for it'll be totally useless to create this kind of map. But it would be okay for you to peek ahead to chapter 21, where we divide life into four quadrants: personal, social, intimate, and professional. So for now, I'd like you to find four sheets of blank paper and a pencil. At the top of each sheet, write one quadrant term followed by the word "goals." For example, one sheet would be titled "Personal Goals," the next "Social Goals," the third "Intimate Goals," and the last "Professional Goals." Select one of these sheets to start, and begin writing down your goals.

As you come up with your goals, be bold and be daring! And be specific. This is the time and place to map out your dreams on paper. Perhaps you'll need to abandon some of your early life goals—like playing shortstop for the New York Yankees—but most of your goals are still out there waiting for you. What are some of your goals for relationships? Do you want to date? Do you want to marry? Do you want kids? *Write it down.* What about social goals? Do you want more friends? Do you want to be a part of a social group or join an organization? *Write it down.* In your career, do you have a dream job? Do you want to go back to school? *Write it down.* Once you've listed a few goals on each sheet of paper, you've completed the first step. Sit down, take a break, and congratulate yourself. This is a great start!

Step 2: List behavioral steps for each goal.

Soon you'll be ready to begin the next phase of your cartography project. For each listed goal, write down the actual behavioral steps you need to take to move toward accomplishing each goal.

Behavioral steps answer the question: What do I specifically need to *do* to address each goal? Behavioral steps help turn goals into reality. Behavioral steps enhance your map by providing you with specific directions. This metaphor makes perfect sense: If you want to drive to someplace new, you need directions. Directions represent the details of how you are going to get from point A to point B.

Let's look at an example: Let's say that one of your objectives on the "Social Goals" page is to "make new friends." To create behavioral steps or directions, you'll need to list exactly what you plan to do in order to meet new people who could become your friends. Here's what the behavioral steps might look like for this kind of goal:

> **Social Goal #1: Make new friends.**
> Behavioral steps for goal #1 (Answering the question, What can I specifically do to meet new people who could become new friends?):
>
> 1. Look in the weekend section of the newspaper or go online to see what activities are happening in my area this weekend that I might be interested in. Select one and attend.
>
> 2. Find out if there is a weight loss surgery support group that I can join.
>
> 3. Contact a local community college and find out what continuing education classes I might be interested in. Select one, sign up, and attend.
>
> 4. Go to a local gym to see if I can work out one day for free to see if I like the gym. Then maybe I could join. This would address two goals: Lose weight and meet people! If I like the gym, join. Otherwise find another gym and repeat the process.
>
> 5. Ask people at work if they know of ways to meet new people in the area. Select one of their suggestions, and do it.
>
> 6. Consider volunteering at a local charity, church, synagogue, food pantry, or community garden. Research my options, select the best one, and start working.
>
> 7. Go to your local community center to see what activities or groups they have available. Select one, join, and attend.
>
> 8. Hang out at your local coffee shop for a few days. Strike up a conversation with someone who looks appealing or

comfortable to you.

Social Goal #2: Enhance my existing relationships.
Behavioral steps for goal #2 (Answering the question,
What can I specifically do to rekindle or strengthen my existing relationships with friends?):
1. Make a private list of five close friends.

2. Select one friend on my list, and write down the top three
   activities that I enjoy doing with that friend. For example,
   shopping, hiking, walking in the park, going to the beach.

3. Call that one friend, and schedule one of those activities
   with him or her.

4. Follow through and engage in the activity with that friend.
   Don't cancel!

Step 3: Just do it.

Notice that all of the behavioral steps listed above are things *to
do*. They involve taking action, engaging in a behavior. Setting your
goals (step 1) is great. Listing your behavioral steps or directions (step
2) is fantastic, and moves you even closer to your dreams. But this
is all for nothing unless you actively pick one behavioral step and
just do it. Making small changes in your actual behavior is necessary to ultimately make big changes in your life. Add these behavior
changes to the thinking changes we've already explored in chapter
12, and you've got a potent mixture for success.

Albert Einstein once said that the definition of insanity is to do
the same thing over and over and expect different results. So if the
way you've been living your life has not led you to accomplish your
dreams, try something else. This same principle applies to taking
action on your behavioral steps. If your first attempt at talking with
someone at the coffee shop doesn't go anywhere, find someone new
the next day. Or try a different approach. Don't give up. You won't
be able to reach your dreams without drawing your map and then
taking clear action to propel your life forward.

Okay, So What's the Holdup?

As you consider driving down the road to the new you, you've made the commitment to give it a shot. You've drawn your map of goals, several in fact. And you've even tried a behavioral step or two to get you rolling down the road. But then you stall, you putter. Something is keeping you from moving forward. You've got your maps, your tank is full of fuel, but you just can't keep yourself moving. What's the holdup?

It may seem contrite of me to say this, but the factor that is most limiting you from accomplishing your goals and dreams is *you*. Before you accuse me of psychobabble shrink talk, let me explain: How you think about yourself and the world is a major factor that could be getting in the way. We've explored this before, but let's look at it a bit closer again.

When you looked at the eight behavioral steps in the social goals list above, did you find yourself saying, "Oh, that won't work!" Come on—tell the truth. Most people tell me that they are very skeptical of behavior change suggestions, either because they've tried some of these things in the past and weren't successful, or because they fear embarrassment or some other discomfort. Some people grew up in a household where they were told "no" or "get real" or "come on, that can't work" to just about everything. You wouldn't believe the number of folks who confide how they were constantly told that what they wanted simply wasn't possible. It's sad, but true.

Instead of saying no, I'm here to ask you, Why not? Somebody has to be the first female president. Somebody has to be the shortstop for the Yankees. Somebody has to be the writer of that next national best seller. Why not you? Why not now?

Interestingly, you'll find that most of the people who are your role models or who have lives you covet are really not smarter, better, more talented or gifted than you. There are a few to be sure, but not many. Think of any great biography you've read. It is more likely that the person had a clear vision of what they wanted and decided that they were not going to let anything get in their way. They were probably encouraged and supported by others, but not always. The key is that they believed they could achieve what they wanted, and that nothing was going to stop them—not fear, not others' beliefs, not other people's objectives. It seems pretty simple in theory, but in practice it's obviously more difficult. Why?

We tend to glorify our heroes as being superhuman. Take Derek Jeter, for example. Sure, he's amazing. All we see is that he makes hit after hit. He must just be naturally gifted, right? Before you turn Derek into a god, consider that this guy has been playing baseball since he was a kid. It's been his passion forever. Perhaps he's got some innate gifts, but I guarantee you that Derek tells everyone that *practice* is the key, not magical talent. Derek is not a god; he's only human. When his professional game goes off track, he works on fixing things until he can improve himself. When his personal life goes off track, he does the same—he works on fixing things until he can improve things. It's what he does. It's what we need to do, as well.

Name any person, go read his or her biography, and I guarantee you that the person has attributed personal success to an unwavering belief in individualized goals and endless hours of practice. So now that you've lost the weight, what's getting in your way? Let's look at a couple of potential roadblocks.

The self-esteem trap.

All those years being trapped in a morbidly obese body may have taken their toll. Most folks have had their self-esteem badly damaged by being 100 pounds overweight for so long. They feel badly about themselves and it's likely that others have made them feel badly, as well. For folks who are obese, weight is often seen as a (if not the) central feature of their physical appearance. Society and the media, which place a premium on being thin, reinforce this view. The end result is a diminished body image, which often generalizes to decreased self-esteem. And the negative emotions associated with low self-esteem sap your power, drain your drive, and do lots to contribute to feeling stuck. Low self-esteem leads to inaction.

On the other hand, some folks are able to avoid evaluating themselves negatively for being morbidly obese. These people recognize that their weight is but one feature of themselves, and they do not allow it to negatively color their overall self-worth. This is a very healthy point of view, and will be of even greater benefit to them after they lose weight following surgery. Consider that you probably never based your self-worth on your eye color. When your self-esteem is healthy, you feel energized, empowered, and motivated to set and act on new goals for yourself. High self-esteem leads to action.

We explored these concepts quite extensively in chapter 18, and you might want to turn back to review the discussion of self-image, body image, self-worth, and self-esteem. The major lesson to learn from all of this is to view your weight as only *one* aspect of your self-image, as opposed to falling into the trap of generalizing your weight to represent your entire self-worth. By limiting the degree to which your weight and size represent your self-image, it's entirely possible to have high self-esteem while being obese.

Another trap than can diminish your self-esteem concerns how you label your problem. There is a tremendous difference between thinking of yourself as "a person suffering with the disease of morbid obesity" and thinking of yourself as "a fat person." The former mindset views obesity as a problem that needs to be addressed. The latter view globally judges the whole person in a vague, negative manner. It's not unusual for this latter view to lead to self-condemnation and low self-esteem. Consider that people with cancer think of themselves as "a person with cancer," not "a cancerous person." As we learned back in chapter 2, there are some clear advantages to viewing obesity as a disease. Shifting your label of yourself to something that can be addressed improves your self-esteem, allowing you to set goals and start taking important behavioral steps. It leads to action.

Your identity prior to weight loss surgery may have been completely based on your weight. When you asked yourself "Who am I?" the answer before surgery may have been "I'm fat." This self-deprecating view may very well be ingrained in your way of thinking about yourself. But with the significant weight loss that comes as a result of surgery, you can slowly chisel away at this global negative view of your self-worth. For more pointers on how to do this, go back and review chapter 18. This is an important step in garnering the energy to set new goals and enact new behaviors, both central to defining the new you.

The fat brain trap.

Feelings of low self-worth are hard to shake. They become quite ingrained and can be slow to change. For this reason, many folks are surprised to find that after losing 100 pounds they continue to feel emotionally as if they are still morbidly obese. It stands to reason that if you've been obese for 25 years, it might take longer than the year or so it took you to lose 100 pounds to adjust. We discussed this concept several times throughout the book already, but it bears repeating: Getting rid of *fat brain* is a lot harder than getting ride of *fat body*.

When you dye your hair or change your hairstyle you probably don't feel like a completely different person. You're still you, but with different hair. Change your nail color, whiten your teeth, get a tattoo, whatever you like, and it still feels mostly like you. For folks whose weight governed their identity, they need to reorient themselves to the world because they feel like they are truly a different person, not simply the same person with a reduced body size.

Losing 100 pounds is more akin to changing your sex or your race. Imagine what it would be like to wake up tomorrow morning and suddenly be the opposite sex or a different race! If your sex were changed, many of the events of your day would be different. Certainly the way people interact with you would be different. Similarly, if your race were changed, you would likely notice some changes in the way you felt and the way others responded to you. Putting it in this context, you now probably understand just how big this change is. For some people it's not just an attribute that has changed, it's their overall identity.

Adjusting to such a radical change takes time. It won't happen overnight. When you move to a new town, it takes a while to adjust and for the new town to feel like home. When you change jobs, it takes a while to adjust and feel like you fit in to the new office environment. When the kids move out, it takes a while to adjust to the quiet. When you have weight loss surgery, it may take time to adjust to almost everything!

Being stuck in your fat brain will naturally slow you down, reduce your motivation, and make it harder to make changes necessary for the new you. Although fat brain may slow you down, it doesn't have to trap you. Using the myriad techniques we've already discussed to tackle fat brain (chapters 14, 16, 18, and 19), you have a fighting chance. Once your brain and body are in sync, the new you will begin to emerge.

Project Me

It's time to focus on you. Think of this as a project no different than building a house or starting a business. It must receive your utmost attention! It's time to stop the excuses, the procrastination, and the delays. You need to make time and focus on rebuilding your life.

This is not always an easy task. There always seems to be something else to distract your attention. Mothers taking care of children, wives taking care of husbands, and some trying to take care of everyone—oh the people pleasers I've met! I cannot tell you how many folks spend all of their energy taking care of others, while all but completely neglecting themselves. This has got to stop. Now it is time to focus on *you*. If not, what was the purpose of having surgery?

This step may require you to let others know that you'll be focusing on yourself for a while. It's time for everyone else to give you some space. You would hope that others would try to help you in this effort, either by assisting you directly or by decreasing their demands on you. But this doesn't always happen. If others know you as devoting all your time and energy to *their* causes, it will be very hard for them to see you shifting some energy to *your* causes. They'll be jealous, personally offended, portray themselves as slighted and hurt, and might even become hysterically wounded and behave as if you abandoned them. This can be hard for you to watch, especially if it's your close loved ones who are behaving this way.

Your first impulse will be to bounce back to your old caretaker self. I am telling you right now: Don't let it happen. Use some of the straight talk skills you learned in chapter 16 to confront these folks. If they truly need your help, let them know that you'll still be there for them, but find others who can chip in so that you don't lapse back to your enmeshed habits. Tell them you love them, and that has not changed and never will. But remind them in your next breath that *you* need a little help now, and that *you* need some space to get better after your surgery. If they don't *give* you the time, you need to *take* the time. Remember, everyone gets only the same precious 24 hours to work with.

With all of this "me" talk, you may think I am moving you in the direction of becoming a selfish narcissist. Not at all! I am simply saying that *now* is the time to ensure that you provide yourself with the attention you deserve, because for too long you held on to the short end of the stick. With time, as you gradually get your life back on track, it will be important to find a healthy balance of taking care of yourself and others.

What if you're one of the folks I mentioned earlier who has very few (if any) people in your support network? In some ways, this can be used to your advantage: There's no one standing in your way. It also affords you the opportunity to make new friends from the ground up. You'll be able to establish new relationships that jive with the new you. Everyone needs social support, and now is the time to make meeting new people a goal. Revisit chapter 14 to learn about making new friends. And when you're ready, hop on over to chapter 15 to explore dating, intimacy, and romantic relationships.

Moving Forward

If there's going to be a new you, you're going to need to be the architect, the chief engineer, and the person that lays most of the bricks on this project. Luckily, you only need two ingredients to build a new you:

1. The firm belief that a *new you* can truly be achieved.
2. The desire to *do* new things, while tolerating some periodic feelings of awkwardness and discomfort along the way.

This is truly why you had the surgery. It wasn't just to be thin. It was to be able to have all of the things that obesity stole from you. So go back to that four-page list of goals, and get busy building the life of your dreams!

Part VI

Moving Beyond Surgery

It's time to move on. This final section envisions the long term, helping you find the right balance of personal, social, intimate, and professional fulfillment and satisfaction in your life. We help you define your version of success, through beneficial strategies that will make weight loss a victorious endeavor throughout your entire life.

21

Restoring Balance

MANY MORBIDLY OBESE PEOPLE LIVE lives that are largely out of balance. Although they might have a good job, some have no social life beyond seeing a few coworkers occasionally after work. They might engage in a solitary hobby (shopping!) that they absolutely enjoy, but it's often hard to find the intestinal fortitude to start dating. Some dimensions of their lives might be going well, but others are falling apart or never really got started.

A balanced life is one where your personal, social, intimate and professional goals are all receiving some quality time. No one is in perfect balance all the time. Life has its twists and turns so that one or another dimension will receive reduced attention from time to time. However, for most people this disparity soon rights itself, and their lives return to balance. If your life is out of balance, it's likely that one or more of these dimensions have been suffering for quite a while.

Your *personal life* includes time spent on individual pursuits such as reading, playing piano, exercising, or simply sitting and staring out into space. It's private time—time devoted exclusively to yourself. Such personal time is immensely important and is probably the

most neglected in today's society. It's during our personal time that
we think, wonder and rejuvenate our dreams and aspirations. Unfortunately, many people think of this as wasting time. Nothing could
be further from the truth! In this case, doing nothing is doing something. Watching the stars in the sky while lying on your back, staring
out on the expanse of the ocean, or looking out your window and
watching the falling snow are wonderful activities. Personal time involves living simply in the moment, which we rarely do nowadays.

Your *social life* is quality time you spend with family and friends. It
can involve vacations, dinners, going to parties, going out to dance,
and the like. Like your personal life, your social life is very important.
Human beings are inherently social creatures, and usually prefer to
be near each other. In fact, we generally find it bizarre for someone
to live alone far away from civilization. We even have a disparaging
term for such a person—hermit. Similarly, we're often leery about
the woman who lives down the hall all alone with her five cats. Being
social seems normal and healthy. Plus modern society now connects
us in ways that were not possible 25 years ago, via online socializing,
e-mailing, chat rooms, texting, blogging, and on and on. We now
have more ways socialize than ever before.

Your *intimate life* refers to time spent with a partner in a loving, romantic relationship. This can include activities such as going to the
movies, day trips, hanging around. It includes time for physical intimacy, as well. While not absolutely essential for survival and often
over-idealized, human beings do seem wired for intimate relationships. Most people want to partner up. Early in life this could involve
casual relationships that blossom into dating. Later in life, whether
marriage or a similar romantic partnership might take hold. Regardless of its form, an honest, romantic relationship is quite desirable
for most of us.

Your *professional life* probably needs little explanation. It represents the time spent working at a job, either out of the house or at
home. These are activities typically related to your profession or professional advancement. If you're pursuing an education, this would
include time you spend in school or doing homework. If you spend
a good deal of your day taking care of your household and family,
then being a homemaker also qualifies. Unless you're the fortunate

recipient of a bottomless trust fund, someone in your household has to work to pay the bills. So the income necessary to support yourself and immediate family is an important aspect of defining your professional life. Finding a job (or jobs) you truly enjoy, or at least one that you more than simply tolerate, is an important part of having a satisfying professional life.

A Balanced Life

In a balanced life, a person feels that life is moving forward productively and that no one area is being wholly neglected, at least not for too long. Folks who live a balanced life know when to shut off their computer and to stop reading e-mails. Being in balance means that you know when to put down that cell phone and spend some time with the kids. You know when to come to bed and share some time with your spouse or partner. You know how to take a moment to just look out the window and relax. You know how to arrange a get together with friends, while asking your spouse to stay home for a night and watch the kids. For most people, a balanced life is the goal to strive for. It looks something like this pie chart:

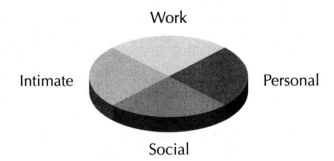

Notice how the four major areas of life are equally represented. Balance means balance: No one part of your life dominates the others. Your overall objective is to live a life where work and play are in alignment. Ideally, you allocate time for work, for friends and family, for your partner, and for yourself. Being in balance means that you are satisfied with your allocation.

There are certainly times in your life where one or another dimension may be diminished, but you can still be in balance. The sizes of these slices of life may shift, like those times you receive a pizza that's not cut to perfect symmetry. Oops—another food analogy! There are people who may not have four even slices of pie, but are still perfectly happy with what they've got. Someone who is retired is a perfect example. This is a person who isn't gainfully employed, but is fully and enjoyably experiencing the other slices of life. Perhaps they're doing volunteer or charity work, or perhaps not. Similarly, some folks are not in an intimate relationship and genuinely prefer it that way. In order to qualify for an unbalanced life, there needs to be unhappiness with how the slices are arranged. Let's explore what an unbalanced life might look like.

An Unbalanced Life

Unfortunately, the world is not interested in our desire to keep balance. Things happen. Our jobs consume us. Our children make demands upon us. Our relationships have rough spots. When the world imposes these pressures, we are sometimes too quick to acquiesce, allowing the balanced equation to come out of alignment. It's not unlike a car having a poor wheel alignment. Things begin to shake and rattle and the tires begin to wear down more quickly and unevenly. Just like with a car, a life out of alignment causes us to shake and rattle and wear down more quickly. Whether we lose sleep, become ill, feel pressured, or become depressed, misalignment takes its toll. Let's look more closely at three common types of unbalanced lives.

The workaholic.

One of the most common types of misalignment is seen in the *workaholic*. We know this person all too well. This is the guy chasing after airplanes to rush home to be with the kids for a few minutes, before leaving again the next morning. He spends endless numbers of hours commuting back and forth to work. When he finally gets home at night, he still has to return all those e-mails. Even weekends aren't impervious to the tentacles of the office. All of those wonderful electronic devices that allow us to be connected so easily also keep us connected when it would be far better to unplug. The workaholic gets swallowed by work and looks forward to weekends,

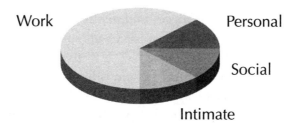

Work   Personal

Social

Intimate

but uses them to catch up on sleep or do even more work. He rarely takes vacations, and when he does he is known for taking the office with him. I've seen just as many women that fall into this category as men.

The workaholic always makes empty promises to his family, to loved ones and to himself. He promises that someday, things will be different. Work will let up and his life will naturally realign. Once he finishes that one project, he can finally relax. But it never happens. A new project is due, work gets busier, responsibilities increase, and time becomes even more precious.

Even if you make millions through all your hours at work, they won't be able to purchase the time lost. I'm reminded of Harry Chapin's song *Cats in the Cradle*, released way back in 1974 but still quite relevant today. In the lyrics, the boy grows up with his father always making promises to spend time with him. But when the father finally has the time, the boy is grown and too busy with his own life to spend any time with his father.

The loner.

The *loner* works all day and spends nights alone by himself. He might have a few friends with whom he corresponds mostly on the

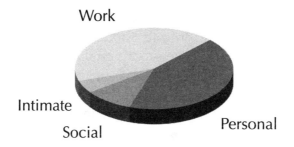

Work

Intimate

Social   Personal

telephone or by e-mail, but he rarely sees them. Maybe he spends some time with family or nieces and nephews on the weekends, but he probably hasn't had the chance to pursue a real intimate and family life of his own.

Anxiety over meeting new people is likely a major concern for the loner. He likely has fears and concerns about intimate relationships and to a large degree has purposely avoided them. Because he spends so much time alone, he is at a greater risk for depression. You can get a better flavor for the personal reality of the loner by revisiting some of the descriptions in chapter 14.

The social butterfly.

The *social butterfly* might be considered the opposite of the loner. Although the loner fears social relationships, the social butterfly on the other hand can't go without them for more than a day or two. She hates being alone and fills her calendar with constant activity, social events, classes and other endeavors. It's very likely that she's not in a meaningful intimate relationship.

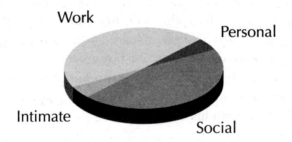

On the surface, the social butterfly may seem happy and content, so you're probably wondering how this could be an unbalanced life. Let me explain. Although this person thrives on social interaction, it is at the expense of other slices of her life. She pursues social contact to an excessive degree, drowning out any opportunity for other pleasures. Instead of a willingness to try out the personal or intimate dimensions of life, she generally avoids them. It's less of a choice and more of a fear of being alone (in pursuing the personal dimension), or a fear of getting too close to someone (in the intimate dimension), or both.

Your Life Portfolio

You may see yourself as the workaholic, the loner, or the social butterfly. Or you may have some other imbalance in the slices of your life. Perhaps you have become the super soccer mom, spending almost all your time on the kids and related activities at the expense of other responsibilities. Or maybe all your energy is being showered on your romantic partner at the expense of developing your own platonic friendships. Regardless of how the slices have been arranged, you're not happy with how things are, and you want to change. So how can balance be restored?

A metaphor you might find helpful is to view your life as an investment portfolio. Most of us are accustomed to the idea of saving money to earn interest or investing money to earn profit. When you're deciding how to invest money, you consider many different types of investments: stocks, bonds, money funds, real estate, savings accounts, cash and a host of other products. Each investment is a different place you can park your money to help it grow.

In the bank of life, instead of investing money, you're investing time and effort. And instead of selecting stocks or bonds, you're selecting personal, social, intimate, or professional areas. The goal is not wealth, but personal fulfillment and happiness. Instead of investing in a stock or bond, you're investing in *you*!

When it comes to investing money, most experts recommend a balanced portfolio. It's not wise to invest all your money in a single stock or a single bond. Likewise, it's not wise to invest all your time and energy in one dimension of life. You need to spread things over all dimensions. Financial experts also tell us that our portfolios need to be reexamined and rebalanced every once in a while, and that we need to consider both short term and long term financial goals. The same is true in the bank of life. Reexamine and rebalance your priorities from time to time. And as you do, set both short and long term goals. You can review some strategies for setting such goals in chapter 20. Isn't it funny how this advice seems obvious and familiar when it comes to our finances, but awkward and oversimplified when it comes to our lives? You might be saying that it just *can't* be that simple. But it really *is* that simple.

Rebalancing Your Life Portfolio

As you've probably figured out by now, most of us have some characteristics of the workaholic, the loner, and the social butterfly. The reasons that we slip into each of these types may vary. Some workaholics have time management problems, and with a little guidance they can be easily overcome. But other workaholics are very anxious about socializing, and they're really loners who work too much. Such issues are more complex, and probably require more work to overcome. Let's turn now to what this work will look like.

Rebalancing the workaholic.

Prior to weight loss surgery, many of my patients identify themselves as the workaholic. It's quite common for a single female patient to admit that because of her weight, she hasn't considered dating for many years, and instead has focused on her career. It makes sense that if one area of your life is too threatening or difficult, you turn your focus on the area that is more rewarding and less anxiety provoking. If working at your job is easier than socializing, you'll probably be spending more time at the office.

For women, the office can become a trap. Without the demands of a family, she has more time to focus on her work and career, and often this effort pays off handsomely. I have seen a number of women who were professionally quite successful. However, anyone in a high-powered career has very little time to dedicate to other areas of life, and goals in these other areas become even further out of reach. I've had the privilege of sitting down with some female CEO's and presidents of companies who have accomplished much in their professional lives, but who also confided that their personal lives were not nearly as satisfying. While this story is not exclusive to women, men generally report that their careers interfere less with their personal lives. Most of the successful professional men that I've seen have been able to marry despite their weight. This probably speaks to the greater bias that our society has against "the big girl" compared to "the big guy," which we addressed in chapter 15.

Many workaholics hold the irrational belief that there just isn't enough time in a day after work to do anything else. If this sounds like you, I would encourage you to consider that how you spend your time is a *choice*. Everyone gets the same 24 hours in a day. No one gets more and no one gets less. How you *choose* to use those 24 hours is what matters. When workaholics tell me that they can't *find* the time, I correct them by saying they choose to not *make* the time. No one gets a 25th hour.

Once the workaholic acknowledges and understands this irrational belief, she can start figuring out how to carve a few hours out of her week to spend time socializing or pursue a loving relationship. You can review some hints on enhancing friend and family time back in chapter 14. And chapter 15 will give you pointers on starting or jump starting that romantic relationship.

Rebalancing the loner.

There are many ways to be a loner, but they all share a common feature: the avoidance of social interaction. Coming out of your shell involves both developing new friends and new romantic partners.

Many patients have said that once their weight significantly decreased after surgery, they began to receive tremendous pressure from friends and family to "get out there" and stop avoiding social interaction. Friends and family are partly correct, for the antidote to being a loner is to find people to be around, either socially or romantically. Each of these dimensions is lacking in the loner's life, and both need to be enhanced.

But this is easier said than done. This avoidance of social interaction does not often occur out of want. Many loners express a desire to be with others, but they avoid the steps necessary to get there. They will avoid social interaction for at least two reasons: an absence of *dating skills*, and a prevalence of *anxiety*. Let's look at each.

As you may remember from chapter 15, there really *are* skills to dating. Sadly because of your weight, you may have never had an opportunity to practice dating—and yes, it requires practice! Now would be a good time to go back to chapter 15 to review and reacquaint yourself with those skills.

If you've had an opportunity to date in the past, you may have experienced a history of rejection on dates due to your weight. And rejection can easily lead you to become shy and withdrawn. With enough rejections in your life, it's not uncommon to always expect the worst, even though you've lost significant weight. This expectation creates great anxiety, and when confronted with the choice of either anxiously dating or calmly being alone, you choose the latter. Your anxiety has turned you into a loner.

For the loner, this anxiety extends to making friends as well as trying to date. Your major concerns are feeling uncomfortable and being embarrassed. You fear that in the presence of others you might act awkwardly and make a fool of yourself. In truth, you may be partly correct. However, once you really get out there, it's rarely as awful as you feared it would be. In fact, it's probably not *awful* at all, just a bit *unpleasant*. And a date where you might have said something that's not perfectly appropriate won't turn into a *disaster*, just a bit *embarrassing*.

I'm choosing my words purposefully, here. I'm trying to teach you to avoid catastrophizing, a common irrational thought process that can make you very anxious and set you up to be a loner. *Catastrophizing* means that you almost always expect the worst to happen. Naturally, if you expect every little white cloud to be an omen for an impending tornado, you'll never leave the house. In fact, your anxiety will paralyze you and you'll never leave the bomb shelter. This is a sure prescription for becoming a loner.

Changing the way you think about your anxiety and reviewing what you're telling yourself about socializing and dating is key to overcoming anxiety. Once you see that there isn't all that much truth to your irrational beliefs, it'll be easier to take that next step and actually get out there and start meeting new people. Add these new thoughts to your behavior skills from chapter 15, and you're ready to roll.

Rebalancing the social butterfly.

The social butterfly is similar to the workaholic in that both need to focus on spending less time on social or work activities, whereas the loner needs to spend more time on social activities. The major problem for the social butterfly is a difficulty with being alone. When she is alone, the anxiety starts to build, and she calms her anxiety by filling her schedule with even more social engagements. This vicious cycle needs to be broken in order to help the social butterfly achieve balance.

The original reasons for a fear of being alone are likely complex, and can vary from person to person. Unpleasant experiences from earlier times in a person's life could certainly be in the mix. Children generally don't like being alone for too long. For many children and adults, even the word "alone" is frightening. Many can't imagine going to a movie or out to dinner by themselves. This problem is often heightened after a divorce or the termination of a long-term relationship where a person doesn't have considerable experience with being alone.

Like with the loner, the general remedy for the social butterfly is twofold. First, you must challenge the irrational beliefs you hold regarding the anxiety or discomfort of being alone. Second, you actually need to practice being alone.

Telling yourself that you "can't stand" being alone or that "I will look stupid eating by myself or going to a movie alone" are examples of irrational beliefs. If you hold such beliefs, they'll likely make you feel awkward and uncomfortable. They might even lead to catastrophizing, as with the loner. How would you challenge such beliefs? Go to a restaurant by yourself for dinner. Take in a movie by yourself. Try it out and see what happens. No one is going to point at you and laugh. At first you might feel awkward, but don't let that stop you. In fact, you might learn that it can be quite enjoyable. There can be great pleasure in shopping alone or doing other activities without the company of others.

Of course being alone all the time is certainly no fun. But did I ask you for that? No! That would be going overboard in the other direction. It's not what I am advocating. Rather, I'm calling for balance: Some time by yourself and some time with others.

We often over-idealize the value of being in a relationship or being around others. Although it's always important to have some social contact, overbooking our social calendar can have its drawbacks. By doing so, we may allow ourselves to be in the company of those whom we'd be better off without. Many people have "friends" who are really only acquaintances. Sit down and take an inventory of all those on your butterfly calendar. Can you really have so many close friends? Do you really need to be in constant contact with everyone who crosses your line of sight?

If you see yourself thinking and behaving like a social butterfly, believing you always need to be around someone, it would probably be useful to look more closely at the reasons behind this need. Do you feel so hopelessly dependent on folks that you can't have a little time away from them? What unnerves you when you are apart? Do you feel too weak to ask for some space? These feelings could be remedied by practicing some straight talk that we discussed in chapter 16.

One incentive to change your butterfly behaviors could be to overcome the feeling that you never get time to unwind. Adding some personal time to your life portfolio can remedy this. Another incentive could be to resolve potential difficulties in the balance of your intimate relationship. I recall having a meeting with the husband of a woman who was complaining that he never spends any alone time with his wife. Time with his wife always involves going out with her single friends or other couples. Clearly the husband felt that folks in the butterfly schedule always seemed to interfere with chances for him to be alone with his wife. This was a problem in their relationship, and striking a new life portfolio balance was necessary to resolve it.

Jack and Jill

The takeaway message from this chapter is that success in your weight loss journey entails striving for balance in the way you construct your life portfolio—the time and effort you spend between personal, social, intimate and professional pursuits. All work and no play can make Jack a dull boy—and one who will likely never find Jill! All play and no work can make Jack professionally frustrated and dissatisfied, and hurt his wallet, too. Our best chance at fulfillment will happen when we endeavor to keep our life portfolio in balance.

22

Success

I T's NOW BEEN A YEAR or more since you've had weight loss surgery. By now you've lost a lot of weight. You probably look and
feel noticeably different than before surgery: You're thinner,
healthier, happier, and stronger. You truly enjoy waking up in the
morning—more than you ever have. So it's time to ask the one tril-
lion-dollar question: Do you consider yourself a success?

As you would expect, the answer to this question is complex.
Success is quite subjective. One person's success can be another person's failure. Success is also fluid. In fact, there's a good chance that
your definition of success has changed since the day of your surgery. Prior to surgery, most folks have truly modest goals for success.
Many simply wish to reduce their risk for future medical problems,
or at least minimize the damage done by existing medical problems.
Most want to improve their physical functioning. But it never fails
to amaze me how these goals become more ambitious as that surgery day fades into the past. As time moves on, folks want more and
more—and why not? It seems only natural to want it all.

Unfortunately, the pursuit of some goals can be a bit like trying
to sail a ship to the North Pole. There are a number of rather nasty

icebergs in the way. It can be quite disconcerting when I speak to someone who has lost a tremendous amount of weight following surgery, has improved her physical functioning, has dramatically reduced her risk for obesity-related medical problems, and looks thinner as well, only to find that she's still unhappy because she hasn't reached some specific objective. What gives?

Taking Stock

If you find yourself feeling unhappy following weight loss surgery, step back and figure out what you're trying to accomplish that leaves you wanting. What's the prize you're after? Did you believe that reaching a specific weight would bring you joy? Were you hoping to fit into a particular size of clothing? Were you hoping to attract people? Were there other goals you were hoping to achieve?

Now would be an excellent time to reassess those ambitious goals you set for yourself in chapter 20. Remember those four lists? You may recall that in addition to creating and pursuing goals, you need to reexamine those goals from time to time. Maybe some goals need to be tweaked. Maybe some need to be modified. Maybe some even need to be abandoned. Stop and take stock. There also may be other barriers that stand in the way of your success. Read on to learn more.

Iceberg Ahead!

As you navigate through the waters of life after weight loss surgery, there are a few common challenges or obstacles to feeling successful. These obstacles are those nasty icebergs I mentioned earlier. The icebergs all share a common ingredient: irrational thought. They all involve how you think about your situation in life, your perspectives on your progress, and your world view. Your thoughts are central to how you feel and behave. Remember: How you think is *everything*.

Good thoughts of the open sea form into icebergs when they become irrational. For many who have had weight loss surgery, the source of these irrational expectations comes from beliefs that were promoted by their family or friends. In some families, a person's weight was a ridiculous focus of attention. For some patients, members of their family continue to express erroneous or irrational opinions regarding the outcome of surgery.

More commonly, the source of emotional upset is from irrational beliefs and expectations expressed by significant others during childhood. Many patients I see prior to weight loss surgery describe painful stories of being emotionally tortured by parents, siblings, friends and others about their weight and eating habits since childhood. When we hear such condemnations over and over, we begin to believe them ourselves.

These irrational icebergs won't melt away overnight. Some take years to go away. And others will never go away. We continue to encounter them from time to time as we sail through life. We've discussed a few irrational beliefs already in this book, such as all-or-none thinking, powerlessness, overgeneralization, and catastrophizing. There are some additional beliefs that can stand in the way of our long-term success, and we'll explore them next:

1. Believing that the number on your scale or the size of your clothing determines your success in life.

2. Trying to achieve the media's definition of size and beauty.

3. Vying for the acceptance of family and friends.

4. Vying for the acceptance of your intimate partner.

5. Telling yourself that you should, must, or ought to.

6. Defining success in absolute terms.

Any one of these obstacles can prevent you from feeling a sense of success and satisfaction from surgery and your resulting weight loss. Let's chip away at each iceberg:

1. The danger of insisting that you achieve a particular goal weight.

Success doesn't come from losing a specific amount of weight. Nor does it come from achieving a certain size of clothing. To prove this point, I can point to several patients who have lost 50 pounds and were happier than other patients who lost over 100 pounds. Isn't it absurd to think that at 173 you're a failure, but at 168 you're a success? Would it be fair to change the names of the women's clothing departments in the store to "Winner's Department" for sizes 0 to 10, and "Loser's Department" for sizes over 10? Of course not! But if you're making yourself upset because the number on the scale isn't quite what you'd like, this is exactly how you're thinking!

What I'd like you to consider is that it's not the number of pounds you've lost that matters. Rather, it's what your newfound "thinner-ness" can do for you. Viewed in this way, success is your ability to accomplish your personal, social, intimate, and professional goals, not desperately vie for some arbitrary number. As you may remember from chapter 18, your weight is only one aspect of your overall self, and a rather trivial one at that.

Allowing weight to dominate your self-image is known as *magnifying* because you're irrationally exaggerating its importance. Isn't it absurd that of all of the ways you can define your self-worth, your weight would be at the top? Not your character, your smile, your friendships, your contributions to society, but that single number? When you think about it, it's utterly preposterous. If somebody told you they thought they were better than you because they had more money, a bigger car, or a more beautifully manicured lawn, you would laugh. It's really no different.

Let's imagine that prior to surgery you weighed 240 pounds and you now weigh 170. But your goal weight was 140 pounds, so you're disappointed. Before you start labeling yourself a failure, ask yourself these questions: Can you now walk more easily than you could before surgery? Are you more comfortable socializing with friends at your new weight relative to the old? Are you better able to fit into movie and airplane seats than before surgery? Can you now more easily perform the duties of your daily life? Has your health improved since surgery? Are you now better able to buy clothing? If the answer to all or most of these questions is yes, you're a success. These are rational markers of success because they represent undeniably real improvements that have resulted from surgery. They demonstrate improvements in your health and quality of life.

Let's think of it another way. You've lost 70 pounds, and now weigh 170, even though your goal weight was 140. You're making yourself miserable and depressed over 30 pounds, despite having already lost 70 pounds? You've lost more weight than you've ever lost in your entire life! You probably weigh less than you have for over 20 years! But you're telling me that you're still upset because you don't weigh what you weighed in high school? C'mon! And you're still lamenting not being able to fit into a size 8 pair of jeans? Isn't that a bit nutty?

2. The danger of believing the media's crazy definitions of size and shape.

I will admit that as a man, it was only during the past few years that I came to realize just how significantly the media's discrimination against obesity disproportionately affects women relative to men. The sad truth is that with all the freedom and prosperity women have fought for and now enjoy, they still remain prisoners of the beauty myth, chained to the false belief that their value is based primarily on appearance. How did this happen and what perpetuates it?

Begin by recognizing that the media acts as a propaganda machine, determined to shake our confidence, remind us that we aren't good enough, we haven't made it, that we just simply don't measure up. If you believe the media hype, it can be quite depressing! In a recent poll in a popular magazine, over 80 percent of women reported that the images of women on television, in movies, fashion magazines and advertising make them feel insecure about their looks. *Eighty percent!* Why is the media bent on making us feel so down about ourselves? Why does the media go to such lengths to make us feel inferior? The answer is quite simple: money.

The media machine is economically driven as billions are spent on items such as cosmetics, new diets, and clothes. This beautifying empire requires us to feel inferior so that we will spend money to feel better. They count on us buying into their myths and misrepresentations. But once we buy, the products simply don't measure up. They don't fall true to their claims. So we listen to more advertisements that make us feel even more inferior. And then we go out and buy even more products. The cycle never ends. The pursuit is endless, the products are endless, the damage to our self-esteem is endless, and the body hatred and damage to our self-worth is relentless and devastating. You never stop the pursuit, falsely believing that you're just one small step away, so you can never really be happy.

Men aren't exempt from this scenario, but it's very different for men and far easier to be an overweight man than an overweight woman. The media's guns are clearly aimed at women when it comes to weight and appearance, although some shots are fired at men from time to time. As I've said back in chapter 18, although there's a place in society for the big guy, there is zero tolerance for the big girl. For example, the leading male character in many television sitcoms can be overweight, but this is rarely the case for the female lead character.

Our shopping culture affects the sexes differently. Men are encouraged to buy technology and electronic toys, which are tangible where one size fits all. Women are encouraged to buy beauty, which is quite abstract where one size absolutely does *not* fit all. Bigger screen televisions and bigger speakers are seen as better. Bigger blouses and bigger skirts are not. In addition, the fashion industry has not always been accommodating to women. Overweight men can purchase virtually identical clothes in larger sizes. You can easily find a nice suit in both size 38 and size 50. Maybe not every suit from every designer, but for the most part, all men's suits look relatively the same. For women, nothing could be further from the truth. Until very recently, designers of women's clothing clearly focused on those who were skinny. Designs that existed in size 6 simply did not exist for size 20. Although the tide may be turning somewhat, the best and brightest in women's fashion are still generally focused on those in the size 2 to 10 set.

WARNING:
OBJECTS IN MAGAZINES MAY BE FURTHER
FROM REALITY THAN THEY APPEAR!

This label should appear on the cover of most popular magazines. The next time you're waiting on the checkout line in the supermarket, take a look at the ten most popular magazines on the rack. The sizes of the women and men on the covers represent about 0.03 percent of the population. The other 99.97 percent don't have a chance to compete, much less measure up. Don't forget that modeling is a career for those that appear on magazine covers, and their eight-hour job is to work on improving their body. Looking good is their profession! Many have had major body makeovers and spend their lives in a gym with a full-time personal trainer. Furthermore, most ads are reproduced, airbrushed or modified by a computer. Body parts are changed at will. These people, as shown, simply do not exist! You're not the freak of nature; *they* are!

Did you know that mannequins can't menstruate? It's true, both literally and figuratively. A major study of mannequins during the 1990's found that most dressmakers' dummies are "genetically unviable." They've got body types—height, weight, breast size, and hip size—that simply don't exist in the natural world. Literally aliens! Unfortunately, it is this impossible, fictitious body image that many women are striving to achieve.

These irrational beliefs are not only coming from advertising. The news networks have jumped on the bandwagon, as well. Why? Because hype equals ratings, and ratings equals money. Every day there are television news segments informing us about how fat Americans are becoming. The typical program shows a graphic display of the skyrocketing rates of obesity, followed by a picture of some children eating corn chips while playing video games, ending with a shot of the rear ends of some heavy people walking in the mall. Then in the very next news segment, they show some starved size zero female movie stars and fashion models giddily chatting at a Hollywood party. What's normal anymore? It's no wonder we're all so irrational and distraught about our weight!

Here's a reality check: What most people think is normal regarding weight is actually not normal at all. Most people do not weigh at age forty-five what they did at twenty-five. Most women that have had several pregnancies do not weigh what they did before those pregnancies. The average American woman is a size 10 to12, not a size 6. In fact, it is these very irrational beliefs regarding weight that contribute to eating disorders among adolescent girls and Hollywood stars. Sadly, these folks are desperately trying to maintain society's ideal, which the human body knows to be abnormal.

3. The danger of vying for the acceptance of family and friends.

Following surgery, many patients are hopeful that family and friends will better accept them, now that they're thinner. Maybe my mother will finally love me now that I'm the thin child that she's always wanted. Pardon the pun, but *fat chance*!

Remember that while you have changed physically, and while you have made many valiant changes in your thoughts and in your behaviors, others around you have not. For them it's been business as usual. Expecting *them* to change because *you* have changed is really asking too much. Chances are if that old crotchety aunt was nasty to you in the past, she'll continue to be nasty in the future. If that close friend was supportive of you in the past, he'll continue to be supportive in the future. The best you can hope for, and should expect, is respect.

4. The danger of vying for the acceptance of your intimate partner.

Many patients tell me that one of the primary reasons they chose to have surgery was to be able to enter an intimate relationship. Some simply refused to date when they were obese, and now are hoping to get out there and land a mate. While the odds may be better now that you weigh less, it isn't a certainty.

If you're already in an intimate relationship, steering clear of your partner's acceptance of you may seem paradoxical. If you were hoping for acceptance from anyone in this world, you'd think it would most certainly come from your closest love. This is very true. But there is difference between mutual dependence on each other, and pathological dependence of one partner on the other. Here we're really talking about the latter.

Some of the problem may occur because *fat brain* takes much longer to leave than *fat body*, a concept we've covered extensively in previous chapters. If your self-esteem is strong and your relationship is healthy, you won't need to desperately vie for your partner's acceptance. But if you're experiencing insecurity about yourself (fat brain still there), even though you've lost a good amount of weight (fat body no more), you could place your relationship at risk by being excessively clingy and dependent on your mate. To deal with these and other challenges of intimacy after weight loss surgery, you might want to revisit chapter 15. In the end, the goal is a balanced acceptance of each other.

5. The danger of telling yourself that you should, must, or ought to.

If you find yourself feeling unhappy following surgery, listen to yourself think. Listen carefully for the words *should, must* and *ought.* Thoughts or utterances that contain these words are called *conditional statements* because you're setting conditions for yourself on how to behave. Are you telling yourself that you *should* weigh 120 or *should* fit into size 4 or *should* weigh what you did many years ago, or *should* weigh what your sister weighs? The flaw in this type of thinking is that this rule is arbitrary. This rule does not appear in the Constitution or the Bill of Rights—maybe in the Bill of Wrongs! It's completely your choice to continue believing these silly rules. Now is the time to get rid of these ridiculous expectations. Reach down along the side of your boat, and cut the nets loose to let those shoulds go.

Let's say it rains on the day that you planned to go to the beach. You might become angry when you start seeing those drops fall from the sky. What you're actually telling yourself is that it shouldn't rain on the day you plan to go to the beach. Isn't it kind of nutty to think that the forces of nature should consult your tanning schedule before deciding whether to rain? That's pretty much what you're telling yourself when you get angry at the rain.

Telling yourself that you *should* now weigh what you weighed in high school is similarly nutty. Your should statement is nothing more than an expression of what you prefer. It's not a legal requirement. It's not a condition of success in life. It's just a preference. Furthermore, it's factually incorrect, given that it's not physically normal to weigh now what you did in high school. When we confuse preferences with irrational rules, we make ourselves terribly upset.

When we get upset that we don't fit into the jeans we wore in high school, or that we don't look exactly as we hoped, or that we have some flabby skin, we can change how we feel without changing our size, weight and skin tone. By telling yourself what you *should* weigh, *should* look like or *should* fit into, you are creating tremendous opportunities to become upset. A better thought would sound something like this: Although I don't fit into the jeans I wore on my wedding day, I look dramatically better than I did 100 pounds ago, and all things considered, that's pretty darn good! Think about how liberating this way of thinking is!

The beauty of endorsing this way of thinking is that you don't need to change the *world* to feel better. Rather, you only need to change the way you *think* about the world. You don't need a new mother, you don't need 27 years of therapy, and you probably don't need to lose more weight. You only need to change the way you *think*.

When you try this new way of thinking, it's normal to feel disappointment. I am in no way suggesting that by thinking in this new manner that you can live a completely blissful life, free from any emotional upset. Disappointment is a fact of life. If you're disappointed that you don't look like you did in high school, or disappointed that you don't fit into those jeans, that's perfectly okay. Disappointment is something we need to graciously learn to accept. Such acceptance will allow you to achieve resolution and move on. By accepting disappointment you are simply telling yourself that it would be nice if the jeans fit; but they don't, and although that's unfortunate, it's not the end of the world.

6. The danger of defining success in absolute terms.

Another irrational thought that can stand in the way of your success after weight loss surgery is called *all-or-none* or *black-and-white thinking*. This type of thinking, which we first covered in chapter 9, creates a dichotomy out of the world: good–bad, right–wrong, pass–fail. Although we know thinking this way is juvenile and ridiculous, we do it all the time.

An interesting example of such thinking is even embedded in the connotation of this chapter's title: "Success." Taken alone, this title implies that you can either succeed or fail. That's nonsense! Success isn't a specific point on a graph. It's not a specific goal weight. It's not fitting into a specific pair of jeans. It's not one good date. It's not *one* of these things—it's *all* of these things, and so many more!

And when you take them all together, you can see that success is best defined on a continuum, like the volume control on your television. Sometimes your success is loud; sometimes your success is quiet; sometimes it is set just right. Success is not like the television's power switch—on or off.

Think about it: How often do things go exactly as planned in life? Who's that lucky? Not me! But unfortunately, this is how many of us think. If you've lost 100 pounds, but aspired to lose 130, wouldn't it be ridiculous to think that you've failed? You're over 80 percent of the way there! In my grade book, that's a B, not an F! Recall what you had hoped to achieve before your surgery. If the surgeon told you that you would lose 100 pounds and never a pound more, would you still have decided to have surgery? Of course you would have. So why isn't that good enough today? Perhaps, it's because you're telling yourself that you've *failed* to achieve some arbitrarily goal (uh oh—a *should!*), whether it be a weight, a jean size or something else.

To overcome all-or-none thinking, some find it helpful to break down your larger goals into smaller steps, like we did in chapter 20. Rather than focusing on global success or failure, concentrate instead on each behavioral step that you're taking in pursuit of those goals. For example, consider the process of applying for a new job. You can't control all the folks involved in making the decision. However, you can control the actions you take in creating your résumé, your cover letter, and your interview. The same applies for personal goals, such as pursuing a new relationship. Rather than obsessing about your overall success or failure in finding a new mate, focus instead on enacting the small steps of dating, like attending a singles event or asking someone out. The Herculean task of finding a lifelong romantic partner suddenly becomes so much easier if you break it down into manageable little steps.

Defining Success

What is hopefully clear from this discussion of irrational thoughts is that in order to *enjoy* life, you need to change the way you *think* about life. A sign in a restaurant near my home reads: "Life is ten percent of what happens to you, and 90 percent what you make of it." Stop and think about that for a moment. It's one of those phrases inside a fortune cookie that seems rather profound for two seconds, but quickly fades from memory by the time you've finished your pineapple wedges. You know those people who have faced unbelievable challenges in their lives, yet always seemed to rise above them? Christopher Reeve comes to mind, among others.

✓ It's not what happens to you that matters.

✓ It's how you respond to what happens that matters.

✓ How you respond depends on how you think.

Changing your thoughts is a challenging, but achievable endeavor. The biggest step involves understanding that how you think is a choice, and acknowledging that it is up to you to change, not the world. When you're able to truly love and accept yourself, despite the fact that you're not perfect, despite the few remaining unwanted pounds, despite that you're not a size six, despite that you've not lived up to the world's expectations, *that* is when you'll know you're a success.

Your Ship's Journey

Imagine that your brain is a ship, how it *thinks* is its rudder and sails, and how it *acts* is how well it cruises through the water. Your objective is to steer the ship toward *your own* destination—not that of your mother, your husband, or your favorite monthly women's magazine. Let them sail their own ships. You need to learn how to get your hands firmly on your own steering wheel so that you can, perhaps for the first time in your life, define *your own* rational goals. Those goals represent your navigational plan, and cover your personal, social, intimate, and professional itinerary.

Weight loss surgery has appointed you captain of your own ship. As you set sail on the open sea, you're excited because you now have more opportunity in your life than ever before. But you also have the responsibility of keeping your ship afloat as you follow your navigational plan, while avoiding that endless stream of icebergs, those irrational thoughts that put your ship in danger.

Do you want to know how to steer clear of those icebergs? Here's the big seafaring secret: Your obsessions with weight and size, the media's endless assault on your body image, and your need for approval from friends, family and significant others are all *completely under your command and control.* Remember, you are the captain! The world may be moving all those icebergs in your path, but you can choose to navigate around them by thinking rationally and behaving responsibly. You don't have to buy into the madness of weighing yourself. You don't need to try to look like the people on television. You don't need your mother's approval. If you can give up those irrational beliefs, there's a very good chance that your ship will stay afloat.

The ship that learns to steer clear of icebergs can traverse oceans. I know you can do it. Happy sailing!

Appendices

Appendix A
Getting Help

WEIGHT LOSS SURGERY IS A major undertaking. As you've seen throughout this book, surgery involves more than simply changing your eating habits. If you've had surgery you already know this. So it's perfectly understandable that you might need some assistance in making all of the behavioral and emotional adjustments that are required to truly be successful. Two questions that are commonly asked about getting help are:

✓ Do I need help?
✓ What kind of help do I need?

Many of the folks I meet during the pre-surgical psychological evaluation have never met a psychologist before. Their contact with me is their first foray into the mental health world. Others have participated in some form of counseling, such as individual psychotherapy, group psychotherapy, or marital/couples counseling. Many have also participated in various self-help options, like Overeaters Anonymous. Some patients come to their initial meeting having taken psychiatric medications to treat depression or anxiety, or are currently taking them. So there's a wide range of assistance that weight loss surgery patients may have sought. Although the above two questions are most commonly asked by people who have never participated in any kind of counseling, it's not uncommon for therapy veterans to still inquire about these concerns.

Before we look more closely at the decisions involved in getting help, it's important to understand the following disclaimer, which essentially says that this book and my advice in this book should never be construed as a substitute for professional care. Here it is. Please read it carefully:

> The contents of this publication are for informational purposes only, and not a substitute for professional medical or mental health advice. The author and publisher disclaim any liability with regard to the use of such contents. Readers should consult appropriate professionals on any matter relating to their health and well-being.

Do I Need Help?

The simple answer to this question is that *you need help when you cannot handle something on your own.* Without question, the greatest obstacle for most people is their own perceived stigma about getting help. When I meet with a patient during the pre-surgical evaluation that has already been in therapy, this hurdle has already been cleared. Understandably, this also adds to my confidence about their chances for success from surgery, because I know that this person is comfortable seeking out help when necessary.

There really is no litmus test that tells you when you need to get help. One way to think about how to answer this question is to revisit what your goals were for weight loss surgery. If you're finding that you're struggling to achieve those goals, or if new issues have popped up that are interfering with your progress, it's probably a good idea to get some assistance.

It's not unusual for someone to seek some assistance *before* they have surgery. I have met a number of folks during the pre-surgical evaluation who concluded through our consultation that there were issues that could potentially interfere with their success from surgery. As a result, they opted to initiate psychotherapy to address these issues *before* those concerns had an opportunity to interfere with their progress following surgery. Knowing that they had professional support available before surgery gave these patients the confidence and solace they needed to proceed with the surgery.

There are a number of reasons why someone might feel the need to seek help *after* weight loss surgery. Many of the issues that you've read about in this book certainly point to such reasons. Here are some examples of the more common problems:

1. Difficulties adjusting to a life that doesn't revolve around food and eating.

2. Difficulties adjusting to being thinner, such as coping with increased attention along with increased expectations from yourself and others.

3. Anxiety related to dating and social relationships, now that you're thinner.

4. Difficulties being compliant with the dietary and behavioral changes necessitated by surgery, such as "eating around" the surgery.

5. Coping with negative reactions from friends, family and others regarding your weight loss.

6. Feelings of anxiety and a sense of feeling lost, now that now that the ultimate goal of losing weight has been accomplished.

7. Coping with feelings of anger towards others who treated you poorly for all those years when you were heavy.

Although these represent the more common problems I see in patients after weight loss surgery, it is of course just a small sample of the larger number of concerns for which folks seek help. Keep in mind that almost any reason is a valid reason to pursue help. If you are not sure, you can always ask at your first consultation with a professional.

What Kind Of Help Do I Need?

When seeking professional assistance, there really is no "best" kind of help. Everyone is looking for something different in the way of help, so you should make sure that you're getting the help you need. All help is not created equal. Also, there is no reason to believe that you need to select only one type of help. For example, many of my individual psychotherapy patients are also taking psychiatric medications, and some are attending support groups. All licensed professionals are trained to keep an eye on the kind of help you need, and they should be able to give you a referral for additional help that they might not be able to provide. If you're not sure, ask.

Without question, there comes a point when someone is getting too much help. Having too many cooks in the kitchen can spoil the broth. But this typically only happens when one cook doesn't know what the other is cooking. This is why it is very important that you let anyone you see know whom else you are seeing, so that your care can be coordinated. That said, having more than one form of help or support is absolutely fine.

Let's look more closely at some of the options for help. The alternatives I list here are by no means the only types of help available. For example, there are quite a few forms of help that I don't cover, such as pastoral or spiritual counseling, many Eastern types of therapies such as yoga, meditation and others.

Bibliotherapy

Perhaps you don't realize it, but you've already taken advantage of what may be the most commonly used form of help: self-help, in the form of reading. In this context, you're a bibliotherapy patient! Millions of self-help books have been published over the years and a number of my patients report that some of these books have made a significant impact on their lives.

Of course all books are not created equal. Some self-help books have been best sellers for many years while others go from the new release table to the discount rack in less than a few weeks. And just because it's a best seller doesn't mean that the advice is good. Be a critical shopper you buy a self-help book. Look closely at the person writing the book. Is it an expert with professional credentials? A person who has actually experienced weight loss surgery? A professional who has experience working with weight loss patients? A writer doesn't have to be everything, but should at least have some experience in the field.

My own bias is for the types of books that ask you to do more than just read. The most effective way to learn is by *doing*, which is why throughout this book I have asked you to make lists and do various exercises to put your new knowledge to work. To get the most out of such books, you really need to pull up your sleeves, dig in, and get to work. You will most certainly be rewarded if you take the time to follow the author's directions. If you read these types of books like a novel without lifting a finger, you'll probably get very little out of them.

In appendix C you'll find a few of my own recommendations for further reading. These were selected for their relevance to folks who have encountered weight loss surgery.

Individual Psychotherapy

Many people refer to individual psychotherapy as "talk therapy." The basic ingredient of individual psychotherapy is indeed talk between one psychotherapist and one patient. However, as you will see, what is talked about can vary considerably. Individual psychotherapy has a number of different "schools," which refer to the approach used by the therapist. Each school ascribes to a different philosophy regarding how psychotherapy should proceed, what the rules are for intervention, and how therapy goals are set. The details of all of this can be pretty complicated. I'll provide a brief overview and you can seek out additional information if you need to know more.

Psychoanalytic psychotherapy is based primarily on the teachings of Sigmund Freud, among others. The general concept is that there are unconscious processes that drive an individual's behavior, resulting in a number of internal conflicts that need to be resolved through the therapy process. In traditional psychodynamic psychotherapy the therapy is generally nondirective and the therapist doesn't speak very much, allowing the patient to guide much of the conversation. The course of traditional psychodynamic psychotherapy can last months or years, with the patient attending sessions several times a week. In more recent forms of this type of therapy, the frequency of visits and the length of the therapy have become shorter. This has occurred in part because of restrictions imposed by the health insurance industry, as well as due to the rise of therapies that have shown equal if not more effectiveness in treating a wide array of psychological problems. One such alternative is cognitive-behavioral therapy.

Cognitive-behavioral therapy (CBT) is a form of psychotherapy based upon scientifically established principles of learning. It's designed to be a short-term, problem-focused therapy. This is not to say that the therapy cannot continue for several months or even more than a year, but the goals of therapy are generally firmly established and progress towards their achievement is monitored regularly. The basic concept behind CBT is that an individual's difficulties have come about as a result of the effects of learning, as well as genetics. The idea is that the patient has learned a set of beliefs and behaviors that have resulted in psychological difficulties. In CBT, the interaction between the therapist and patient is quite active. The therapist is one part teacher and one part coach, and is an active partner in the treatment process. The therapist doesn't allow the treatment process to unfold. Rather the therapist helps direct it with the patient as an active participant. The patient can expect to complete homework, which would likely involve writing down thoughts and feelings and completing behavioral exercises.

As an example of CBT, consider a patient who has lost a great deal of weight but now has high levels of anxiety in social situations. Although the patient is thinner and feels better about her appearance, she continues to feel very awkward and shy in the company of others. Plus this anxiety is greatly interfering with her goals of dating and making new friends. The objectives of CBT would be to help reduce the client's anxiety, and to help her socialize more often and with greater comfort. The patient would work with the therapist to understand what irrational thoughts and behaviors contribute to the anxiety, and then help her change these irrational thoughts and behaviors to promote improved socialization.

The patient would be asked to practice entering social situations and to document what thoughts she was experiencing that could contribute to her anxiety. Similarly, she would be asked to perform certain behaviors while socializing, and to resist performing other behaviors. For example, the patient would be encouraged to approach others, talk to them, and make good eye contact. She would also be instructed to avoid looking away from others, hugging the walls, and avoiding conversation. The therapist would help assign exercises and help the patient learn or relearn how to socialize and be more comfortable, while the client would be responsible for doing the assigned exercises and reporting back to the therapist on progress.

CBT treatments have been found to be effective for a wide range of problems, including anxiety, depression, eating disorders, sexual dysfunction, and personality disorders, among others. As I'm sure you've figured out by now, my philosophy and the one that guides this book is cognitive-behavioral. There are a number of other schools of individual psychotherapy, including *Gestalt, interpersonal,* and *systems,* among others.

Group Psychotherapy

Group psychotherapy is simply psychotherapy conducted with a number of individuals. Group sizes can vary, but many experts believe the optimal number of participants is between six and ten. Less than six participants, and you don't get much of a group process going. More than ten participants, and it's hard to create an atmosphere where everyone feels like they're able to contribute and get something out of the process. Just like with individual psychotherapy, the philosophy of group therapy can follow any school of thought.

People sometimes choose group psychotherapy over individual psychotherapy because they enjoy the process of group therapy. Another reason is that group therapy is generally less expensive than individual therapy. There is also a strong argument to be made that some psychological problems are better suited to group treatment over individual treatment, particularly where social support or constructive confrontation might be indicated. Group therapy is also great to address problems that involve social contexts, like social anxiety or performance anxiety. What could be better than working on your public speaking anxiety in front of others? Similarly, a group focused on a specific topic can be very conducive to problem solving, because everyone in the group struggles with the same types of challenges.

Support Groups

Support groups provide participants with support and encouragement in a group environment. But support groups are generally not considered to be a form of treatment for psychological problems. Support groups are not group psychotherapy. While such groups may be run by a professional, the professional is not providing psychological treatment like you would see in group psychotherapy. This is especially true when someone who is not a mental health professional is conducting the support group. I am making this distinction because if you're experiencing significant psychological distress, at least one form of help you receive should be from a licensed mental health professional. A support group is a fine addition to such treatment, but is often inadequate as the only form of help because the group leader is rarely trained or qualified to address significant psychological problems.

Support groups generally focus on addressing issues relevant to the overall group, and do not focus on resolving issues that any particular group member is having. When group sizes exceed 20 people, it's simply impossible for a weekly or monthly meeting to efficiently treat the issues of an individual group member. In fact, in some support groups it's very easy for you to not utter a word, so you are really only learning information through observation and not participation.

There are support groups for just about anything. Certainly there are weight loss surgery support groups, but there are also single mother support groups, divorced men's support groups, shopaholic support groups, and on and on. The only thing needed for a support group is a gathering of people, a common issue to discuss, and a meeting place. In fact, if seven women go out for drinks after work and they all talk about issues relating to their job, you've got a workplace support group!

Support groups are fantastic for allowing people with a common concern to get together and express their difficulties, and receive guidance from others coping with similar concerns. Oftentimes, relationships form between members of the group in a manner that is often discouraged among members of group psychotherapy. If you're experiencing some difficulties following surgery, I strongly encourage you to attend at least one support group meeting in your area. Many patients have told me that attending support group meetings after surgery was one of most helpful strategies to enable them to remain focused on getting better.

Online Support

Online support is becoming an increasingly popular method of assistance, and can play an important role in your journey after surgery. Such support generally comes in the form of blogs, video programs, or chatting. Such support often allows you to ask and answer questions from others who have had or plan to have surgery. On occasion it's possible to get support from professionals on some sites, as well. As is the case with live support groups, online support should not be the only form of help you receive if you believe that you are experiencing significant distress.

It's important to be a little wary of online information because it can be difficult to know whom you're really speaking to. It can also be hard to evaluate the credibility of information you're receiving. You've got to be a critical consumer, knowing that the quality of information can vary tremendously from source to source. Nevertheless, many of my patients have told me that chatting with people online was helpful because they were able to get support and information on demand, without having to wait for formally scheduled groups at their local hospital. In addition, it can provide you with a greater measure of anonymity that doesn't exist when you attend a support group in person. But be careful because nothing you do online is ever totally anonymous, though it can be confidential.

Psychological Medications

It is certainly beyond the scope of this discussion to provide detailed information about every psychiatric medication. However, I can say that medication can be quite helpful for folks who are experiencing significant levels of anxiety or depression, or are struggling with an eating disorder. For many, the biggest obstacle is getting past the perceived stigma of taking medication for a psychological purpose. Taking medication for depression, anxiety or any psychologi-cal issue doesn't mean you're "crazy." Similarly, taking medication doesn't mean that you couldn't handle things on your own.

Many of my patients have used medication as a tool in conjunc-tion with psychotherapy and support groups to help them get their lives back on track. Sometimes a mental health professional will sug-gest you consult with a psychiatrist to evaluate whether medication would be right for you. It's especially important to consider medica-tion if you're finding that psychotherapy and support groups alone are not helping with your distress. Although many medications do have side effects, these need to be weighed against the potential ben-efit of lowered distress.

One place to start is to have a conversation with your primary care doctor. If your doctor is comfortable prescribing medication, this is one possibility. Another option is that your physician may refer you to a psychiatrist or psychopharmacologist for a consultation to discuss your situation and determine if medication is appropriate. If you're presently seeing a mental health professional, you could certainly discuss the possibility of taking medication. Most psycholo-gists, social workers and other mental health providers have rela-tionships with psychiatrists, so it shouldn't be difficult to receive a referral.

Appendix B
Worksheets

IN THIS APPENDIX YOU'LL FIND three worksheets designed to put some of the ideas discussed in the book into practice. Each worksheet will help you learn more about yourself. Ultimately the goal is to help you understand and work through some of the thoughts, feelings, and behaviors that surround your cravings for food, weight gain, weight loss, and alternatives to eating.

- ✓ The *Cravings Diary Worksheet* will help you identify the triggers that prompt your urge to eat. You'll find information about how to use this worksheet in chapters 7, 8, 10, and 12.

- ✓ The *Eating Alternatives Worksheet* will help you generate and try new adaptive behaviors that serve as a healthy alternative to eating. It's discussed in chapter 7.

- ✓ Finally, the *Diet Trials Worksheet* will help you evaluate the successes and failures you've had with past weight loss attempts. It's use is described in chapter 11.

Cravings Diary Worksheet

Document as much information as you can that relates to factors that trigger your urge to eat. These urges to eat are called "cravings." Sometimes the urge occurs due to hunger. Other times the urge is triggered by something else. When you learn to identify the triggers for your cravings, you will become better at controlling your urges to eat. You also will learn how to change what you eat and engage in activities other than eating.

Date & Time	Where am I?	What food do I want?	What food am I actually eating?	What am I doing? With whom?	What am I thinking?	What am I feeling? What mood am I in?
December 15, 8 P.M.	Den.	Chocolate covered peanuts.	Nothing yet.	Watching television alone.	This television program is mediocre.	Bored and lonely.

Eating Alternatives Worksheet

Document your efforts to practice alternatives to eating when you experience cravings. When you have an urge to eat, keep track of what you tried to do instead of eating, and whether this method helped you overcome your craving. Sometimes it will; sometimes it won't. By trying different alternatives to eating, you will learn that you don't have to succumb to your cravings. More importantly, you will develop new and healthy habits.

Date & Time	Where am I?	What am I doing? With whom?	What am I thinking?	What am I feeling? What mood am I in?	What did I do instead of eating?	How did it go?
December 19, 9 P.M.	Den.	Watching television alone.	I want potato chips.	Bored and lonely.	Went out for a walk with my neighbor.	Pretty well! I had a nice time and forgot about the chips.

From *Through Thick and Thin: The Journey of Weight Loss Surgery*
© 2012 by Warren L. Huberman. All rights reserved. Published by Graphite Press.

Diet Trials Worksheet

Keep a log of your most recent attempts to diet. Dieting is difficult, and diets rarely work. But by dissecting your motivations surrounding your past diet attempts, and by conducting an honest assessment of their success or failure, you'll develop a better understanding of the circumstances that stand in your way of maintaining a healthy weight.

Date Diet Began	Date Diet Ended	For How Long Did I Diet?	Why Did I Start Dieting?	Why Did I Stop Dieting?	How did it go?
January 1	February 15	Six weeks.	It's the beginning of a new year, and I want a fresh start.	I was starving almost all the time! And I felt irritable. It felt like forever to even lose a little bit of weight.	Not too well. After I got off the diet, I actually weighed more than when I started. I felt like a failure.

Appendix C
Further Reading

Roth, Geneen. *When Food is Love.* Penguin, 1993. 224 pages.

An excellent resource for exploring the food–mood connection and how emotions can affect and disrupt eating.

Craighead, Linda W. *The Appetite Awareness Workbook.* New Harbinger Publications, 2006. 200 pages.

A very hands-on workbook that encourages the reader to learn about the cognitive, emotional and behavioral factors that affect their eating. The book requires the reader to document their eating behavior along with thoughts and feelings and to begin making significant changes in their behavior.

Fairburn, Christopher T. and Wilson, G. Terence. *Binge Eating: Nature, Assessment, and Treatment.* Guilford Publications, 1993. 419 pages.

A comprehensive book designed primarily for professionals who work with patients with binge eating difficulties. Current research findings in binge eating are thoroughly reviewed. This book also offers interesting insights for the layperson. Factors that contribute to the rise and maintenance of binge eating are explored and treatment options are reviewed.

Fairburn, Christopher T. *Overcoming Binge Eating*. Guilford Publications, 1995. 247 pages.

An outstanding and user friendly book for both laypersons as well as professionals. Dr. Fairburn reviews the literature on binge eating and dispels many misconceptions about what binge eating is and is not. The book also includes a self-guided treatment program for binge eating, including many useful worksheets to assist in the process.

Ali, Khaliah, Lindner, Lawrence, Ren, Christine C., Fielding, George T. *Fighting Weight: How I Achieved Healthy Weight Loss with "Banding," a New Procedure That Eliminates Hunger—Forever*. Harper Collins Publishers, 2008. 256 pages.

This terrific book explores Khaliah Ali's journey from obesity to gastric banding surgery and beyond. The book includes a detailed explanation of Ms. Ali's weight loss struggles and the process she experienced throughout the weight loss surgery process. Very useful for the reader who is strongly considering gastric banding surgery and wants more information about the process from start to finish.

Kurian, Marina S., Thompson, Barbara, Davidson, Brian K., Roker, Al (forward). *Weight Loss Surgery for Dummies*. Wiley, John & Sons, 2005. 352 pages.

An extremely user-friendly book written by a surgeon and other professionals that work closely with surgical weight loss patients. This book explores almost every conceivable aspect of weight loss surgery including deciding if you are a candidate, medical and emotional issues related to surgery, paying for surgery, eating after surgery, returning to work, and plastic surgery. An invaluable resource for the reader who wants to know about all aspects of weight loss surgery.

Schiraldi, Glenn R. *The Self-Esteem Workbook*. New Harbinger Publications, 2001. 200 pages.

If you are wondering whether there's a way to improve your self-esteem, this might be a good place to start. Weight loss surgery can provide you with many benefits, and feeling better about yourself is certainly one of them. But there are no guarantees. If you are looking to enhance and tweak your self-esteem, consider this book.

Author Biography

W ARREN L. HUBERMAN, PhD. is a clinical psychologist and clinical instructor in the Department of Psychiatry at New York University School of Medicine. He is an affiliate psychologist at the NYU Langone Medical Center and at North Shore LIJ–Lenox Hill Hospital. Dr. Huberman is a consulting psychologist to the NYU Langone Weight Management Program, and has been since its inception in 2000.

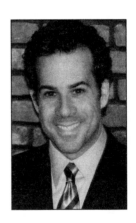

Dr. Huberman specializes in behavioral medicine, with an emphasis on health behavior change and behavior modification in the areas of weight loss, stress management, and the treatment of anxiety and mood disorders. He maintains a private practice in psychology with offices in Manhattan and Rockland County, New York.

Dr. Huberman is also president and founder of the Performance Consulting Group, LLC, which helps individuals and organizations enhance the performance of top executives and senior managers. His work has been featured in medical and mainstream publications, and he has appeared on national television and radio.